Living Fit entails a lot more than simply diet and exercise. Balance is the key to walking a straight line and it is also the key to living a straight life toward the goal of pursuing a more healthy you. Read this and reap!

O. S. Hawkins
Bestselling author of *The Joshua Code*
and the entire Code Series

Living Fit is a fantastic heaven-inspired GPS that will transform your life. It's loaded with life-transforming wisdom keys.

Mike Evans
1 *New York Times* Bestseller

Ronnie Floyd is a wonderful mixture of pastor-teacher and empowering leader. For as long as I've known, he's lifted up the people around him. In this book, he has given us a helpful resource with the tools you need for fit living, a lifestyle he has modeled consistently for many years. Pick up a copy for yourself and for a friend, and discover the steps you can take to living a life that counts.

J.D. Greear, PhD
Pastor, The Summit Church, Raleigh-Durham, NC

Holy, healed, and healthy people change the world! In *Living Fit*, my dear friend Ronnie Floyd provides a Christ-centered, Bible-based plan that will empower you to do just that live fit in every aspect and shine for Christ!

Samuel Rodriguez
President NHCLC
Lead Pastor New Season
Author of *Be Light*

Relevant and inspiring. Pastor Floyd gives key perspective on how to make the most while living here on earth. In *Living Fit*, he unlocks the secret to ignite a more connected life and a healthier you. His step-by-step, biblically backed guide is easy to follow and convicting to implement.

Shelley Simpson

Execu̶   ̶ Commercial Officer
President Hignway Services at J.B. Hunt Transport, Inc.

Having seen thousands of pastoral transitions, I'm convinced that living a balanced life is the one key difference between finishing well and crashing and burning. Dr. Floyd has.done an amazing job of living in balance, and has now given us a roadmap that will help all leaders finish well. Read *Living Fit* today. It could make all the difference.

William Vanderbloemen
Founder and CEO
Vanderbloemen Search Group

Want to live life to its fullest? My friend Ronnie Floyd shares in *Living Fit* what he has learned and what he lives. To be healthy and whole and reach the potential to which God has called us, we must attend to the fitness of our body, mind, and soul.

Tony Perkins
President, Family Research Council
President, Council for National Policy

There are no compartments in our lives that God doesn't say, "Mine!" He desires to use our body, soul and spirit for His great compelling purposes. Thanks Ronnie for pointing us to an intentional pathway to see that He does!

Kathy Ferguson Litton
Director of Planter Spouse Care
North American Mission Board

Of the thousands of books written and published each year, very few are *must read* material. *Living Fit: Make Your Life Count by Pursuing a Healthy You*—without a doubt—is at the top of that first-class list. Robust, hearty living is yours when you apply vital principles of five prescribed topics encompassing spirituality, finances, physical attributes, emotional well-being, and relationships. Join me in reading, applying, and growing through the book's content for making our lives count more for God and man.

Gil Strickland Sr.
Founder and Ministry Ambassador
Marketplace Chaplains
Exceptional Employee Care

If there's anyone who has mastered the art of balancing life's never-ending demands, it's Ronnie Floyd. Leading a life of impact demands we care for every minute of our days and every inch of or bodies, minds, and souls. *Living Fit* is the fruit of decades of living purposefully. It has timeless wisdom for us today and for generations to come.

Jack Graham
Pastor of Prestonwood Baptist Church
Founder of PowerPoint Ministries

Ronnie Floyd has struck one of the essential truths about what it means to live a truly healthy life: giving the proper care and attention to every part of our beings. *Living Fit* will reveal the areas of your life that have been neglected and provide you the necessary tools to build habits that lead to a successful and fulfilling future. If you want to know what it takes to find spiritual, physical, relational, financial, and emotional success, this is the book for you.

Dr. Tim Clinton, Ed.D., LPC, LMFT, BCPCC
President of the AACC

According to tradition, the philosopher Socrates said, "The unexamined life is not worth living." Christian, know life is a precious gift. Because you are made in God's image, your life has incredible potential and ought to be lived well, intentionally. In *Living Fit*, Dr. Ronnie Floyd explains how to make this a way of life. Get started getting fit now by following the practical steps in this strategic book.

Jerry A. Johnson
President and CEO
National Religious Broadcasters

Ronnie W. Floyd

LIVING FIT

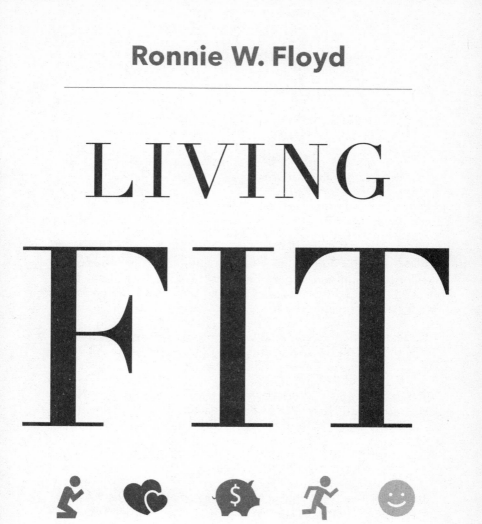

Make Your Life Count
by Pursuing a Healthy You

PUBLISHING GROUP
NASHVILLE, TENNESSEE

Dedication

I am dedicating this book to my seven grandchildren, praying God will create in each of them the passion of Living Fit.

I love you, Peyton, Reese, Parker, Beckham, Jack, Norah, and Maya.

Always remember: I love you more!

One Thousand Thank Yous

One thousand thank yous to the following people who have contributed to *Living Fit: Make Your Life Count By Pursuing A Healthy You*:

- Gayla Oldham and Melissa Swain, for their work of editing and proofing this manuscript.
- Brian Dunaway, Director of Communications at Cross Church, who has helped me think through this book and its message as well as the communication aspects of it.
- Our incredible Cross Church Communications Team, for their assistance in creating the cover of this book and formulating a strategy to communicate it with the world: Andrew Albright, Miguel Gamboa, Tori Lasater, Clayton Lyon, Mary Michels, John Phillips, Betsy Puckett, and Denise Smith.
- My literary agent, Robert Wolgemuth, and his gifted associate, Austin Wilson, and the entire team at Wolgemuth and Associates.
- Johnnie Moore, Jonathan Williams, and the entire team at The Kairos Company.
- Devin Maddox, Taylor Combs, and the entire team at B&H Publishing.

- My friends, Jeremy Roberts, Ben Mayes, Jeff Crawford, and my son, Nick Floyd, who joined me in the initial meetings for this book.
- My Staff Team and my beloved Cross Church Family, for their willingness to share their pastor with others.
- My wife, Jeana, who gives me away by hours and sometimes days during seasons of writing.

I could never make this vision walk without your help.

Contents

Section 4: Living Fit Financially

Section 5: Living Fit Emotionally

Introduction

You have only one shot with your life. Make it count.

Life is a gift from God. You do not determine how long you will live, God does.

As for me, it's a sobering thought to realize that even before this book is on the shelf, I could die.

Yet, I also know that while I cannot determine how *long* I will live, I can determine how *well* I do live. Right now.

For over a decade, I have had my annual physical checkup at the world-renowned Cooper Clinic in Dallas, Texas. This process is extensive and takes a few hours. But, it is also very thorough, needed, and helpful.

The Cooper Clinic is interested in the whole Ronnie Floyd, not just the physical body of Ronnie Floyd. From my first appointment there, this was more than apparent.

They taught me the importance of monitoring the various gauges in life that further my personal health and wellness. From their evaluation of my answers to the questions I complete annually, all the way to extended time with my personal physician, they talk to me about every dimension of my life, not just one part of it.

Every question challenges me to measure how I am doing in various parts of my life. I could be tempted to give the doctors the answers I think they want, but I am forced to honestly stop and gauge these various parts of my life. This helps the professionals navigate to a fuller understanding of what the hard data tells them about the condition of my body. And my life.

Of course, it's routine for them to assess the hard data. From my heart rate to blood pressure, to the results of my stress test to my blood work, these results do not lie. Then, of course, there is the hands-on physical part of my annual check-up. I will spare you the details. You know how these things work.

This continual process year after year has inspired me to prepare for the writing of this book. A by-product of the experience at the Cooper Clinic is that I have an elevated understanding of gauging, measuring, and assessing my own life . . . in every area.

This leads me to today. I'm so eager to share with you what I have learned, not just from the last few years, but also throughout my entire life, about what it means to live fit.

As you can imagine, writing this book calls me into extreme accountability. My resolve to live this way has become part of the permanent record, and I am hereby giving you permission to speak up if you hear that I have failed to live up to these standards.

This book is not a complete presentation that gives to you all the answers and ways to live fit. But it is an intentional action I am taking to create a conversation that is long overdue.

If you want to join me on this journey, come on. Let's continue this conversation not just throughout the book, but also beyond. Let's begin.

Living Fit: Make Your Life Count by Pursuing a Healthy You will help you learn to read your life's gauges accurately today.

Living Fit will identify each area of your life and give you direction for living healthy tomorrow . . . spiritually, physically, relationally, financially, and emotionally.

Living Fit will equip you to check each gauge in your life that measures how you are doing in these critical areas.

Living Fit will motivate you to put together a winning plan that will become your ongoing strategy for true and complete fitness in every strategic area of your life.

Living Fit will reveal the importance of your mind, will, emotions, and body being under the authority of God's Spirit as it becomes mightier and controlled daily, consistently, and regularly.

> Your choices today will determine your fitness tomorrow. Choose now for your future to be fit.

Each choice you make will lead you toward or away from a healthy you. Your choices today will determine your fitness tomorrow. Choose now for your future to be fit.

God Wants You to Live Fit

Your life *will* count when you develop a winning plan and remain focused and intentional about following it.

I believe this book has the capacity to condition you to be able to win in your life, make it count, and have a clear direction for your future.

We do not need to be like the guy who kept a hammer on the front seat of his car. When one of his dashboard gauges flashed an annoying warning like "Service Engine Soon" or "Low Fuel," he would pick up the hammer and smash the gauge. Who needs this kind of interruption and aggravating distraction in life? I have places to go, people to see!

Of course, this is silly. No reasonable person would do such a thing. Why? Because those gauges are there for a reason. They communicate helpful and potentially life-saving messages—information you and I need to know.

Gauges are instruments that measure significant markers. This is true in your car, in airplanes, and in your life.

Sadly, sometimes you and I go through the normal routine of our schedules and never take the time to check each personal gauge to see if we are strong in the moment and heading toward a healthy tomorrow. When we are too preoccupied with life to check on our gauges or when we don't like what we see, we become like the guy taking the hammer and smashing the gauges on his dashboard.

Discernment helps us wisely and objectively judge the importance of checking our personal gauges, and it trains us to check each one consistently. Discipline helps us take action when one of these gauges tells us something needs to be changed. These steps will lead us to get fit for today and stay fit for tomorrow.

The Bible is God's book for life. When the Bible speaks, God speaks. God says this to us: "Let us lay aside every hindrance and the sin that so easily ensnares us. Let us run with endurance the race that lies before us" (Heb. 12:1). God's Word calls us to put away anything in life that hinders us from being all God wants us to be. For the Jews, it was their Levitical system that was contradictory to the claims of the gospel of Jesus Christ, which has once and for all fulfilled the requirements of that system. Just as any runner in a race will strip away any piece of clothing that will weigh him down and hinder his performance, we must remove anything in life that keeps us from being all God desires us to be.

Some Bible translations use the word *weight* instead of *hindrance*. In the original language, this word means . . . weight. This refers to anything that keeps you from running the race well.

Look at it this way: You can run a race if you're a hundred pounds overweight, but you're not going to win. You can climb a mountain trail smoking a cigarette, but you may end up in a wheezing heap before you reach the summit. You and I can ignore the messages our gauges are sending us, but the outcome will not be pretty.

Why would we choose not to pay close attention to our life's gauges and operate our lives at the highest level? Why shouldn't we have an extreme commitment to check each gauge in life and then determine to live with the highest commitment to success in every dimension?

> You and I can ignore the messages our gauges are sending us, but the outcome will not be pretty.

Do you want to navigate to a healthy tomorrow? Do you want to be fit in every way so you can live your life at the highest level and make the greatest impact possible? Do you want a plan to win?

Then you must again see what God says to us in His Word. He says, "So I do not run like one who runs aimlessly or box like one beating the air" (1 Cor. 9:26). As the apostle Paul articulated these words under the leadership of God, he stated that he did not want to run his race in the Christian life as some athletic runner who ran with uncertainty or without direction. In fact, he indicates that no serious runner would do this.

Paul continued by stating he did not want to run his race with God like a boxer who trained endlessly and never entered the ring. Rather, he wanted to engage with all he had to be all God wanted him to be.

You see friend, living the life God wants you to live is the greatest opportunity you have. It isn't easy, but it's worth the hard work and training required to win.

By the time you conclude this book, you will understand the biblical significance of being fit. You will also recognize the specific areas of life that need to be continually evaluated. I also believe this book will provide a great motivation for you to take the needed actions to be wholly fit.

How You Will Live Fit

I am going to share the strategy for you to live fit through five sections in this book. In each section, there will be four chapters that are long enough to communicate clearly, but short enough to be crisp and to the point. Then, I will conclude the book with a final motivation for you to be on your way to a healthy you.

This holistic approach will prepare you to live fit in a balanced way. Not just because it is a good thing to do, but because it is the biblical, spiritual, and right thing to do, guaranteeing—as far as it depends on you—you will live an impactful life.

Section 1: Living Fit Spiritually

The first section of the book deals with living fit spiritually. This is the most foundational and most important area in which to live fit. While some Christians make the mistake of thinking this is the only area we should pursue fitness, we are right to place the highest priority on living spiritually fit. As your spiritual life goes, so goes the rest of your life.

Section 2: Living Fit Physically

God's desire is for us to see our whole person set apart for God so that we can live fully. Therefore, we must not only focus on our spiritual fitness; we must also be committed to being fit physically. Through discipline, orderliness, reasonableness, and awareness, we can glorify God in our physical bodies.

Section 3: Living Fit Relationally

The importance of healthy relationships cannot be overstated. God has created us to relate to Him personally and to other people relationally. Living fit relationally demands us to die to ourselves daily and live selflessly, to love others unconditionally, to connect to other people, and to follow Christ's example of service.

Section 4: Living Fit Financially

Financial troubles create enormous pressure in life. These challenges drain you emotionally and completely distort your vision. Money is important and it is integrally connected to our wisdom, responsibility, generosity, and the legacy we will leave after we are gone. Jesus said, "Where your treasure is, there your heart will be also" (Matt. 6:21). Let's pay careful attention to our use of money.

Section 5: Living Fit Emotionally

We are created as emotional beings. Your spiritual fitness, physical fitness, relational fitness, and financial fitness will affect your emotional fitness. God desires for you to live a complete and full life in every way. This is only possible when you are emotionally whole. You must realize that one part of your life is not disconnected from the other parts of your life. Emotional health requires a holistic approach.

Set Your Sails

When you determine to live your life in a healthy way spiritually, physically, relationally, financially, and emotionally, it is like taking a long voyage through troubled waters. Your enemy, Satan, will do all he can to take you under. His aim is to create a very unhealthy you that operates in dysfunction.

This is why you must set your sails toward your destination of being *FIT,* and determine with all you have and all you are that you are going to become healthy in every area of your life. When you do this, you will be on your way to living fit and becoming a healthy you.

Let's begin the journey now.

SECTION 1

Living Fit Spiritually

CHAPTER 1

Live Purposefully

There have been times in my life that I have struggled with my own identity. I have felt the pressure that I must have a title or assignment to feel significant. There were times in my younger years where I struggled with not living in a metropolitan region of America. I felt reduced. I felt insignificant. I felt like others did not recognize the value of where I served.

At times, this created a discontentment that was unhealthy. While the struggle was real, it became apparent that it doesn't matter what anyone else thinks relating to these kinds of things. What matters is that you know and live out God's purpose for your life. When you choose to live out God's purpose for your life, while titles and assignments and opportunities are nice, you will find joy and happiness regardless of the specifics, because you are living purposefully.

Recently, we conducted a professional survey with our entire church. In order to do this, we allocated ten minutes in each of the eleven Sunday services on all five of our campuses. One of the many questions we asked our congregation that day was the following: *What topic would be of most interest to you during a*

Sunday sermon? We received responses from several thousand people.

Through the years, we have not conducted very many of these surveys, but we are very passionate to create ways to hear from our church members and find out where their needs are. We are here to equip the saints to do the work of the ministry. If we do not know what their needs are, we cannot know how to equip them most effectively. That is why we asked this specific question. Here is what we learned.

Other than teaching through books of the Bible, as I have done regularly through the years, there were two topics people asked us to address: *finding purpose* and *marriage.*

Needless to say, we have exhausted this survey to learn all we could about the uniqueness of our people and their personal needs. As we listened to their interests, we began to discuss how we could address these needs, one of which was finding purpose.

You cannot live fit spiritually if you do not live purposefully. Without purpose, people live aimlessly. I have become convinced the need to live with purpose is greater than the survey may have revealed. People want to know their life matters.

Four Declarations

Therefore, in this chapter, I am going to give you four dynamic statements about purpose. I want you to think of them as declarations. When this chapter is finished, you will have four declarations that will empower you to live purposefully. You can declare these in prayer daily, but you can also declare them as a testimony to other people, to the world, and even to Satan, who always wants to distort our purpose. I promise you, this will really help you, as it has helped me.

The first declaration about living purposefully is . . .

Declaration 1: I believe God has a purpose for my life.

One of the most well-known passages in the Bible is Romans 8:28-31. It says:

> We know that all things work together for the good of those who love God, who are called according to his purpose. For those he foreknew he also predestined to be conformed to the image of his Son, so that he would be the firstborn among many brothers and sisters. And those he predestined, he also called; and those he called, he also justified; and those he justified, he also glorified. What then are we to say about these things? If God is for us, who is against us?

This section of Scripture amplifies this reality: *I believe God has a purpose for my life; therefore, I am living with purpose.* How do we know this?

The word *predestined* is used in Romans 8:30. It means to decide beforehand or to predetermine. I believe that according to Romans 8:29, predestination is grounded in the foreknowledge of God. God knows everything from the beginning to the end; therefore, He knew before and He knows today who will be responsive to His call to salvation. As God set His pursuit toward those whom He knew would respond to His call to salvation, He sovereignly called us into a relationship with Him, endowing us with a purpose in life. Everyone God called into salvation is now set free from all sin, and God looks at us as though we had never sinned, all because of His abounding grace toward us. Upon our death, God will glorify us, freeing us for all of eternity from the power and penalty of sin.

> You are living purposefully—whether you feel it now or not.

Therefore, unquestionably, biblically, and theologically, you should know that you are living purposefully—whether you feel it now or not. You can declare with all confidence to everyone: *I believe God has a purpose for my life!*

Now that we understand more clearly some of this section, go with me in a further, deeper look, that is much more practical for your life. I think it will be encouraging to know . . .

God Is at Work in Your Life

Yes, God *is* at work in your life. Did you know that Romans 8:28 informs us that in each and every part of your life, God is at work? These things work together or cooperate to produce a greater effect than they could individually. God works through all things in concert together.

God is always orchestrating everything in your life to work together for your benefit. He sets His heart toward all of us who love Him intimately and pursue Him passionately. God's intention and will is always good and always best for you.

I have to stop and qualify this, because it is very important for us to understand. ***Everything that happens to you is not good, but God uses everything for your ultimate good.***

Not everything that happens to you is good. At times, we are affected by the poor choices we make. Other times, the sinful choice of someone else can influence our lives dramatically. Some examples of this could be a husband who is unfaithful to his wife, leading to a divorce that impacts every person in the family. Another example would be business partners affected by someone in the partnership that goes bankrupt and a domino effect occurs, cratering not just one person, but several. While everything that happens to you does not seem good, God uses it for your good and for His glory.

The great news is that God is absolutely sovereign and He shapes us through everything we face in life. Yes, God has a purpose for everyone who loves Him. Be encouraged because God is always at work in your life, for your good. God is always moving you to walk toward His eternal purpose of being like Jesus.

> God is always moving you to walk toward His eternal purpose of being like Jesus.

Our God who knows everything from the beginning has also predestined us to be conformed to the image of His Son, Jesus Christ. God is fashioning each of us into the image of Jesus. When we experience spiritual rebirth, God puts us into His family and sets His purpose into our life.

Regardless of who you are, where you are, or what you do in your life, if you are a Christian, God is always moving you to His eternal high purpose: *Making you more like Jesus Christ.* He created you to live your life with God's purpose always on your mind, becoming like Jesus Christ.

The only way you will ever feel fulfilled is to know that God is always sovereignly and lovingly using everything in your life to make you more like Jesus Christ, for His glory.

God Is Always for You

Romans 8:28-31 is powerful in every way. In fact, Romans 8:31 proposes a question: "What then are we to say about these things? If God is for us, who is against us?" Walk the rest of this day and week knowing that God is always for you! I believe God has a purpose for your life because God is always for you.

Keeping all these things in mind will help us understand our value, identity, and future. Therefore, I must warn you about something very important.

Caution: *Your identity and future cannot be determined by a job, a title, or any human achievement.*

If you attempt to define yourself by a job, a title, or some human achievement, you are on your way to experiencing an enormous disappointment, possible depression, and guaranteed purposelessness. If it takes any of these things to give you identity and purpose, you are in trouble, because life is always transitional and temporal. Your purpose is far greater than a job, title, or human achievement. Your purpose is to be like Jesus Christ.

Therefore, you can declare unashamedly and convincingly: *I believe God has a purpose for my life.* Living purposefully will make you more fit spiritually and it will provide much greater clarity as you navigate your way to a healthy you.

Standing on this declaration leads me to share a second declaration with you.

Declaration 2: I will pursue God's purpose for my life.

How seriously do you take your spiritual life? Resolve now that you will pursue God's purpose for your life with great intentionality.

After God watched His people sin, which led them to spend seventy years under God's judgment in a place called Babylon, He gave them another chance to pursue His purpose for their lives. Even after their second year in Babylon, God used Jeremiah to encourage them that even after disobedience and judgment, they could begin, right then, to pursue God's purpose for their lives.

Jeremiah 29:11 says, "'For I know the plans I have for you'—this is the LORD's declaration—'plans for your well-being, not for disaster, to give you a future and a hope.'" This is a positive word from God, given through Jeremiah, that could shape them for the rest of their lives.

The Lord was so gracious to them that He led them to call out to Him in prayer and seek Him with all their heart. He was confident they would return to Him, because His purposes never fail, and He had a purpose for their lives. God used even this season of judgment for their good and for His glory.

Whoever you are and whatever your current circumstances, pursue God's purpose for your life. Through every season of your life, from good to bad to mediocre, pursue God's purpose. Now and in the future, pursue God's purpose with a great expectation that God is working in your life, believe Him for your future with hope.

Intentionally pursue God's purpose for your life. Conversationally—as with a trusted friend—talk to God about His purpose for you and your life. Passionately seek God with all your heart, knowing He will fulfill His purpose for your life. Expectantly believe God will renew you by living purposefully. Pursue God's purpose for your life.

Declaration 3: I believe nothing can hinder God's purpose for my life.

I'm sure you are familiar with the story of Job in the Old Testament. In a brief period of time, this wealthy and prosperous man lost his possessions, his children, and his health. His wife told him to curse God, and his closest friends betrayed him, saying that all these bad things were happening to him because he must be living in sin.

Yet, we know that what his friends said about him was not true. The Scriptures say that Job was a man with complete integrity who feared God and turned away from evil. He was regarded as the greatest man in the East, rising very early each morning to worship the Lord his God.

Even after these life-altering and devastating experiences, Job declared with great confidence these words in Job 42:2: "I know that you can do anything and no plan of yours can be thwarted."

When Job testified that no plan or purpose of God could be thwarted, Job was saying there is absolutely no purpose or plan of God that can be clipped off, cut off, withheld, limited, restrained, or eliminated by anyone or anything!

Everything that happens to you is not good, but God uses everything for His ultimate good in your life and for His glory. He is always moving you toward His likeness.

Even as it was for Job, it will be for you. Life is not easy; it is full of challenges and even some losses. Job deeply believed what we need to believe: *I believe nothing can hinder God's purpose for my life!* He trusted this because he knew God could do anything. Do you? While some people may experience a level of restoration as Job did, others may live to the end faithfully yet lose their lives as mentioned in Hebrews 11. For both groups, the ultimate promise is that God's eternal purposes will come to fruition.

> The way you view God will determine how you view everything else in your life, including your problems, challenges, and even losses.

The way you view God will determine how you view everything else in your life, including your problems, challenges, and even losses. Because Job so believed this, his future became meaningful, productive, and fruitful again.

Please understand this clearly—what God wants to do, He will do. God is unstoppable! Therefore, each of us should declare this personally: *I believe nothing can hinder God's purpose for my life!* Yes, God *is* able! He *is* unstoppable!

Declaration 4: I will serve God's purpose in my generation.

What will you be known for in your life? How will you choose to live between your birth and your death? How will you impact your generation?

These are important and powerful questions we need to take seriously.

Personally, I want to be known as King David was at the end of his life. Acts 13:36 says, "For David, after serving God's purpose in his own generation, fell asleep, was buried with his fathers, and decayed." Here is the bottom line according to this text: After David had done the will of God in his generation, he died.

God determines our length of time on this earth. We do not. I have lived long enough now to see young men that I loved dearly, who followed God passionately, die suddenly and tragically. To this day, I just do not understand. But here is what I do know: God determines our length of time on this earth. Therefore, I believe when we have served God's purpose in our generation, we die.

While God determines our length of time on this earth, each of us resolves what to do with the time He gives us. Choosing how you live and what you do with your life between your birth and your death is your decision. What I do know is that God wants each of us to live purposefully.

What purpose does God have for you in your generation? Are you serving God's purpose in your generation? Discover why you are here on this earth. Then, live it out purposefully.

In summarizing this chapter, you have been called to live purposefully. This is critical to being spiritually fit and pursuing a healthy you. Each day in prayer to God, begin to make these four declarations about living with purpose. I believe it will increase your faith, enlarge your vision, and impact the world around you.

Wherever you are reading this right now, if possible, say aloud these declarations of faith about living purposefully.

Declaration #1: I believe God has a purpose for my life.

Declaration #2: I will pursue God's purpose for my life.

Declaration #3: I believe nothing can hinder God's purpose for my life.

Declaration #4: I will serve God's purpose in my generation.

Friend, you are now on your way to a healthy you. Live purposefully. People who live with purpose change their world.

CHAPTER 2

Live Dreaming

The process always precedes the product. When my eating is healthy and my physical fitness is productive, I feel better. I even believe I look better! Therefore, the process always precedes the product.

Many times in life, we are not pleased with the results we are getting. Being displeased with the results may be all we see, but the greater reality lies in the process that led to these results. If we want a different product, we must evaluate the process and adjust it as needed to obtain the results we desire.

Just as this principle is true in business, sports, or any realm of life, it is also applicable in our spiritual lives. Being fit spiritually ignites you to dream about how God wants to use you to deeply impact your world. Your vision for your life will never be any greater than your faith, and your faith will never be any deeper than your daily walk with Christ. The more fit you are spiritually, the greater the possibilities that await you in the future.

This is where the value of the process is deserving of our personal evaluation. Being fit spiritually cannot and will not occur if we do not live intentionally. The more intentional we are about deepening our daily walk with Christ, the more likely we will become fit spiritually. This leads to a growing realization that God desires for us to live freely. Freedom is not the power to do what we want, but the power to do what we ought. This freedom occurs as we permit God to remove the shackles of our past sins and mistakes, which in turn leads us to experience an inner spiritual cleansing and health that is imperative for us to become what God desires. When this occurs, we begin to live purposefully. This empowers us to believe again that God has a purpose for our lives and nothing can hinder the purpose of God for us.

Therefore, how intentional are you daily in developing your spiritual walk with the Lord? Are you living so free from your past that you are experiencing an inner spiritual cleansing and health that has been refreshing? Are you living out your faith with a clear and compelling purpose in your workplace, your home, and as you are just living life?

> The more fit you are spiritually, the more clearly you will hear God's voice and realize He wants to use you to make a difference.

If you can answer these questions in the affirmative, it's likely you are in a spiritual posture to believe that God wants to use you in ways He has never used you before. The more fit you are spiritually, the more clearly you will hear God's voice and realize He wants to use you to make a difference. The bigger the difference He makes in your life daily, the greater the impact you can make in every way.

Keep this dream alive!

This Is What I Am Talking About

God has exploded our church's outreach to college students. Each semester, I walk into a worship venue on our Fayetteville

Campus located just a few minutes from the University of Arkansas. Even though we have to do two worship services each Wednesday night due to limited parking and the size of the room, these students keep coming. When I stand to speak to these college students—ranging from six hundred to one thousand, depending on the time during the semester—there is something that really fires me up.

By the time you are reading this, our Fayetteville Campus will have been relocated near Interstate 49, no more than four minutes from the University of Arkansas. This new, sixteen-acre site with plentiful parking and a larger worship venue will open possibilities to reach an even greater number of college students, not just on Wednesday evenings, but in our Sunday worship services.

When I spoke to these students recently, I determined as I prepared that I would approach my time with them with a different perspective. I returned to what leadership guru John Maxwell taught me years ago. John always talks about ways he can add value to the people he speaks to and meets with. While I have always tried to keep this in mind, as I prepared to speak to these college students, I focused on how I could add the greatest value to their lives. I wanted to give them something specific they could remember and do for the rest of their lives.

If you have never had the privilege of speaking to hundreds of college students at one time, there is nothing like it. When I look at their young faces filled with so much promise and their hearts bursting with vision, I humbly want to help shape their dreams and their futures.

This is what I am talking about. I want to encourage them to live dreaming—not just living their dreams, but God's will for their life and future. I want them to believe that God can do anything, anywhere, with anyone—including them. I want each of these students to believe God can do more in a moment than any of them could ever do in their lifetime.

Yes, I want these college students to live dreaming. Regardless of your age or place in life today, I also want you to live dreaming—not just dreaming about what you want to do, but what God may want to do in and through you in your life.

Part of this dreaming is exactly what this book is about. My challenge to you in this book is to become fit—spiritually, physically, relationally, financially, and emotionally. This holistic experience is a process of navigating your way to a healthy you.

Live Dreaming . . . It Will Add Value to Your Life

While the Bible is full of stories about many great men and women of faith that would have added value to the lives of the college students I spoke to that night, I determined that God was directing me to go with one particular story of a man with whom they would be likely to identify.

Regardless of your age, I believe you will identify with this man also. He was just a normal guy. His name is not listed in God's "Hall of Faith" as noted in Hebrews chapter eleven, but I really believe he may be given a special place in heaven one day.

When I read his story years ago, it added value to my life. In fact, it still does. I know it added value to hundreds of college students that night when I shared it with them. I am convinced his life story and practice will add great value to your life.

In 1 Chronicles 4, name after name is listed. Among this long list of people whose names are not familiar to us, we read about a man named Jabez. While only two verses mention his name, what is said about him has shaped the prayer life and future of millions of people.

Jabez had a painful past. In fact, 1 Chronicles 4:9 states, "Jabez was more honored than his brothers. His mother named him Jabez and said, 'I gave birth to him in pain.'" His mother named him what she named him because when she had him, it was evidently a more painful childbirth experience than she had with her other children.[1]

While we do not pick up in this passage that Jabez had major issues with his brothers like Joseph did as noted in the book of Genesis, we do learn that Jabez was more honorable than his brothers. From this brief reference, Jabez was worthy of respect and even influential with his brothers. Perhaps he wanted to be more and do more for God than his brothers. We do not know specifics, nor do we want to presume to, but regardless, he was set apart from his brothers.

With a name like Jabez, he could have cried "Foul!" and lived like a victim, but he didn't. We need to do just as he did. *We never need to permit the pain of our past to become the destiny for our future.* This is not God's will for any of us.

This is a dream to live out daily and a dream to keep on dreaming. It will not only excel your faith, but it will also propel your life forward to be all God wants it to be. Live dreaming this dream because it will add value to your life and future.

Most people have a level of pain in their past and face ongoing pressures in their daily lives. You and I do, too. Each of these shapes us into being more of who God wants us to be.

Talk to God about Your Dreams

Why should you live dreaming? Why should you talk to God about your dreams? The more fit you are spiritually, the more deeply and widely God will impact your world. This is why you should live dreaming. You should talk to God about your dreams and let Him create some God-sized dreams in you that He desires to see done through you and in the future He has planned for you.

Do as Jabez did. He prayed, and God answered. Enough said.

First Chronicles 4:10 says, "Jabez called out to the God of Israel: 'If only you would bless me, extend my border, let your hand be with me, and keep me from harm, so that I will not experience pain.' And God granted his request."

Take the Bible for what the Bible says. It says, "Jabez called out to the God of Israel." After he prays briefly, the Bible states: "And God granted his request." He prayed. God answered. Enough said.

We need to talk to God about our lives, our dreams, and our future, just like Jabez did. While his words do not become a simple formula for success, they do show us how we need to talk to God about our dreams.

Jabez was a convictional man. He cried out to God for help in his future. He prayed with intensity, passion, and in humility, but with great conviction. Jabez knew who to talk with about his dreams and his future and even how to talk to Him. He talked to God.

> Call out to God about your dreams and your future. I believe if you do, He will fill your life and future with His dreams.

Who are you talking to about your dreams and future? Your friends, family members, colleagues, or even some headhunting firm? Call out to God about your dreams and your future. I believe if you do, He will fill your life and future with His dreams.

What I am about to share with you comes directly from God's Word. It is not a recipe or a hoop to jump through in order to get God's future for you, but it is God's Word that you can stand on for your life and your future.

Four Ways You Can Talk to God about Your Dreams

From God's Word in 1 Chronicles 4:10 and the example of Jabez, let's talk about four ways you can talk to God about your dreams.

1. Lord, bless me.

When you ask God for His blessing upon your life, you are asking God to place His favor, His grace, and His power upon you. You are asking Him to intervene in your life supernaturally. Just as Jabez prayed fervently, you should do the same. Just as Jabez knew that he needed the blessing of God upon his life, surely you know the same.

Therefore, ask God for His blessing upon your life, your dreams, and your future.

2. Lord, extend my border.

While Jabez desired what was seemingly more land, this meant his influence would become greater. Just as Jabez did not let his present or future be dictated by what appeared as borders or obstacles, neither do we.

Therefore, call out to God to extend open doors for your life and future, where your influence for Him could be increased and extended for His glory. This is not about us having more of anything. It is about believing God wants to use us to make a greater difference for Him. Since we believe that God has a purpose for our lives, we also believe He wants to give us dreams for our future that will open doors so we can make a greater difference for Him.

3. Lord, let your hand be with me.

Jabez knew he needed the power of God and His guidance through his life and future. You see, just as Jabez experienced God opening doors and extending borders, he needed more of God's power upon his life. You might ask how I know this. The Bible says that God granted his request.

Never apologize for asking God to place His hand on your life and the dreams He has given you for your future. As God opens the doors for your future, you are in greater need for His power for your life.

4. Lord, keep me from harm.

Jabez knew that as God blessed him, he needed God's protection. Not just from Satan or other people, but from himself. He did not want to be harmed, nor did he want to harm others. This is a great lesson for each of us. We must ask God to protect us from evil, but also to protect us from ourselves each day.

Believe God, Live Dreaming

Prayer is the bridge to your future—not just for your life today, but for the future life God has planned for you. He wants to deposit dreams into your life that only He can bring about.

When you live spiritually fit, you are getting your life into a healthy position for God to do great work through you.

Pray fervently. Keep your motives pure. There is no telling what God may choose to do in and through you. Believe God. Live dreaming.

God can do more in a moment than you can ever do in a lifetime. Therefore, determine now: *I will live spiritually fit.*

CHAPTER 3

Live Freely

We are broken. Our distance from God is immeasurable. We are not just disconnected from God, we are disconnected from people. Therefore, we feel we are alone as we walk through life.

We are insecure, overwhelmed at times, with a sense of worthlessness. Failure seems to be fatal. Guilt never leaves us. Shame seems serial. Pain is perpetual. Life is a burden.

Knowing we do not measure up, we manipulate ourselves to spend most of our time trying to win the approval of others. We quickly discover this is a treadmill race to nowhere, but we often stay on the treadmill anyway.

We feel bound. Trapped. Dead inside. Hopeless.

But then, God comes. Mercy begins to wake us up. Hope rises like the sun on a clear day.

Someone connected with me, telling me a story about a man named Jesus who came to heal the sick, wake up the dead, forgive sins, and set each person free.

I listened. I opened my heart. Something happened to me. The one telling me the story said it also happened to him.

Jesus saved me. Changed me. Set me free.

Today. Tomorrow. Forever.

Free.

As I began to hear stories about Jesus, what had just happened to me began to make sense. One time when Jesus was sharing His message of freedom, many believed in Him. Then Jesus told them something profound: "You will know the truth, and the truth will set you free" (John 8:32). He then went on and said it with even more force and conviction: "So if the Son sets you free, you really will be free" (John 8:36).

Now I know why I feel like I do. Jesus set me free. Not just free, but really free.

The Journey to Being Spiritually Fit

As we journey together on this path to being spiritually fit, you may need to stop reading and pull away to spend some time in personal reflection and examination. Since you are reading this book because you desire to be fit spiritually, physically, relationally, financially, and emotionally, this is not only a good thing to do, it is imperative. I want to lead you through accepting, releasing, and experiencing some things. Let's learn what it means to live freely.

Accept

When you desire to accept Jesus Christ into your life, you have to receive some realities about yourself and Him. Sometimes accepting realities about situations is easier than accepting realities about yourself.

I believe one of the reasons people struggle with being healthy spiritually is because they have never accepted some realities about themselves. This is why I want us to pull aside for a few moments. It all begins here.

Accept Responsibility for Yourself and Your Sinfulness

Each of us struggles to accept responsibility for ourselves and our sinfulness. Our pride blinds us from seeing the truth. Therefore, we rationalize our choices and often blame other people and situations. These actions prevent us from living fit spiritually and being healthy inwardly.

The curse of Genesis 3 still plagues you and me today. We are sinners by our nature, having inherited the guilt of Adam and Eve, and we are sinners by choice. Just as Adam and Eve chose sin, we choose sin. Just as they blamed others for their poor choices, we do the same thing today.

As I said, we do this because we do not accept responsibility for ourselves and our sinfulness. We need to accept what we read in Ephesians 2:1-3: "And you were dead in your trespasses and sins in which you previously lived according to the ways of this world, according to the ruler of the power of the air, the spirit now working in the disobedient. We too all previously lived among them in our fleshly desires, carrying out the inclinations of our flesh and thoughts, and we were by nature children under wrath as the others were also."

> Each of us struggles to accept responsibility for ourselves and our sinfulness.

Before Christ came into my life, there were times I felt dead. I felt bound, trapped, and held captive by a power bigger than me. I wanted to do the right things consistently, but I never could. The very things I did not want to do, I ended up doing. And the very things I wanted to do, for some reason, I could not do them.

There is a reason for all of these things. I was dead spiritually. There were moments when I fell from where I knew God wanted me to be. I missed God's mark for my life horribly and continually. I wondered then and still periodically wonder even now, why? Here is the short answer: I was living in and out of Ephesians 2:1. I was dead in my trespasses and sins. I was trapped, held captive by sin, by a power bigger than me, by Satan. I was living in and out of Ephesians 2:2. I was carrying out actions in order to satisfy my personal desires and inclinations. Even with the pleas from others and God Himself, I continually kept turning away from God. Yes, I was living out of my own selfish desires and sinful nature.

Finally, I stopped rationalizing my poor choices and blaming others. As the Holy Spirit began to convict me of my sinful nature and sinful choices, I stopped running. I was under immense conviction. Playing church nauseated me. I got sick and tired of playing church games. But then things changed.

As I reflect upon that season of my life, I still get mad at Satan and even madder at myself. Since sin ruled me, my actions were stupid. Sin did not just affect my life; it dominated my life.

No one but me is responsible for any of these things. I own them today, and I had to own them then in order to deal with them when God began to convict me. Knowing what I know now makes me regret the choices I made then. But today, I accept responsibility for myself and for my sinfulness.

Perhaps you need to do as I just did. You may need to go back and take full responsibility for yourself and your sinfulness. You were just like me, dead in trespasses and sins. While it may not have been pretty then and it may not be pretty now, own it. Take responsibility for it. It is imperative in order to become fit spiritually and healthy inwardly.

Accept the Claims of the Gospel of Jesus Christ

Earlier in this chapter, I wrote these words: *But then things changed*.

What changed? My life and yours, before we met Christ, were written about clearly in Ephesians 2:1-3; then everything changed.

It changed through the words written in Ephesians 2:4-5, "But God, who is rich in mercy, because of his great love that he had for us, made us alive with Christ even though we were dead in trespasses. You are saved by grace!"

"But God" is one of the greatest phrases in the New Testament. Jesus changed everything. He changed me. Has He changed you? If Jesus has changed you:

- When did He change you? Perhaps you cannot remember the day nor the hour, and you may question it at times, but you believe He did change you.
- Where did He change you? If you are a genuine follower of Christ, you may not remember the day you met Christ, but you will never forget the place where Jesus changed your life. If you cannot answer this question, you may really need to come to Jesus now and let Him change you today, wherever you are right now.

There is nothing like meeting and knowing Jesus Christ personally.

My life changed when Jesus Christ came into it. When He did, every sin was forgiven and my future for all of eternity was settled. I came to a point where I had to accept who Jesus claimed to be and what He claimed to do when He lived on this earth.

When I was helpless and hopeless, His mercy found me. I deserved hell; He promised me heaven. I deserved to die in my sins; He removed all of them. On that day when I met Christ personally, I did not understand it all, but I have a greater understanding today. He loved me so much that He pursued me and awakened me by His Spirit, drawing me to experience salvation and a personal relationship with Him. Since that day, I have never wanted to go back to what it was like before I met Jesus.

I have been saved by grace. I did not work for my salvation, but it was given to me freely. And I received it with a grateful heart.

Jesus lived a sinless life on this earth. He suffered beyond what we can humanly imagine. He died a cruel and horrible death. He was buried in a tomb. On the third day, Jesus was raised from the dead. After appearing to many as the resurrected Christ, He ascended to heaven and today is exalted at the right hand of God. One day He will come again for His church. Forever we will be together with the Lord. These are the claims of the gospel of Jesus Christ.

> I did not work for my salvation, but it was given to me freely.

As I repented of my sins and turned by faith to Jesus fully and completely, I was saved by grace. This is the power of the gospel of Jesus Christ.

What Jesus did for me, He will do for you. While our stories are different, the result is the same. Jesus changed our lives.

Therefore, I can live freely, because while I accept responsibility for myself and for my sinfulness, I know that these sins are no longer held against me. I have been put into right relationship with God by His grace. How can I not accept the claims of the gospel of Jesus Christ?

I appeal to you to take responsibility for your own sinfulness. Then accept the claims of the gospel of Jesus Christ. Living fit spiritually will never happen until you do.

Release

When we choose to live under the guilt and shame of our past, it rocks our present and limits our future. The longer I follow Christ and serve His church as a pastor, the more I see the reality of wrecked lives. Our enemy, Satan, always points people to the past, while Jesus, our Lord, heals our past and points us to the future. If we know Christ personally, we need to walk away from the past toward the future God has for us. Being set free means we have been liberated from our sin and past. Jesus came to set us free and release us to the future.

I want to challenge you to release these things today.

Release Past Sins

When you receive the gift of grace into your life, you are provided salvation from all sins: past, present, and future. So

> When we choose to live under the guilt and shame of our past, it rocks our present and limits our future.

many Christians live with enormous guilt and condemnation from their past sins. It is important to read and live your life by Romans 8:1, "Therefore, there is now no condemnation for those who are in Christ Jesus" (NIV). While Satan, your flesh, and the world want to drag you down, God wants to remind you that you are set free from all sin and condemnation.

Therefore, release all of your past sins. Do not go there. While the scars from the choices you made in past sins will always be there, Jesus has released you from the penalty of them, as well as their dominion over you and your pleasure in them. You are released . . . live like it!

Release Past Mistakes

Releasing your past mistakes in life is critical to the future God has for you. Being saved does not mean we never make mistakes. We do, and plenty of them!

You and I have bought things we should never have bought, said things we should never have said, watched things we should never have watched, and gone places we should never have gone. This does not mean these are all sinful acts of rebellion against God. Some mistakes are just what they are—mistakes!

Our judgment should have been better in the moment of decision-making. When cause and effect kick in, it is what it is. A mistake! We make mistakes and oftentimes, while they may not be sinful, we have to live with the reality of cause and effect. Regardless, release your past mistakes.

Release Present Challenges

Everyone is dealing with some present challenges. I can name mine. What about you?

These present challenges we face should call us to go to God in prayer and seek truth and wisdom from the Bible. Prayer and direction from God's Word will see us through.

Therefore, pray about your challenges. Add them to your daily prayer list. Talk to God about them. When you read the Bible, see what He may have for you relating to these challenges. Then release your challenges to God daily. Surrender them to Him one by one.

I appeal to you to release to God your past sins, past mistakes, and present challenges. Living fit spiritually is impossible if you are not willing to release these things to God.

Experience

Now we are ready to experience all God has for us. Why? Being set free from the bondage of your past and your present challenges leads to experiencing inner health spiritually. Remember where we are and what we are doing: *Pursuing a healthy you!*

Being fit spiritually is so important to your future. This cannot occur living in the past and in condemnation. God wants you to live freely. When you have worked through your past and released it to God, you are ready to experience all God has for you.

Why choose guilt over grace? Shame over strength? Pain over healing? Failure over success? God has released you from those things. Let them go!

God accepts you. God loves you. God is faithful to you. God wants to connect with you.

God wants you to experience inner health spiritually. He wants you living in the limitless grace of God. Learn from your past. Be free to live your future. Prepare to become all God wants you to be. This is living free.

CHAPTER 4
Live Intentionally

As your spiritual life goes, so goes the rest of your life. As you look at the dashboard of your life and check your spiritual gauge, what lights are flashing? What are you learning about your life right now? This instrument is vital in helping you measure where you really are in your walk with Jesus Christ.

Your spiritual life will never outpace your intentional commitment to prioritize it in your life daily. Your deliberate commitment to walking daily with Christ is imperative to your spiritual success.

The development of your spiritual life impacts every area of your life. You cannot delegate your spiritual development to anyone else. It is impossible! This is up to you to do completely.

Over Christmas break during my college years, my brother asked me to build a barn for him. He is a much more gifted carpenter than I, but he was trying to help me out. Even though this was not in my skill set or passion, I needed the money. I was able to accomplish the task, but the barn did not stand the test of time. In a few years, the barn began to lean and eventually became unsafe. My brother would've been better off to build the barn himself than to delegate something to me I was not able to properly do.

Just as this was not a wise decision relating to a barn, we cannot expect someone else to build our spiritual lives for us. A barn is one thing, but no one can construct your daily walk with God. It has to be intentional, purposeful, and personal. It is up to you.

You have to realize this: *God desires to have a meaningful relationship with you daily.* With Him, you are never put on hold and you never have to stand in line. He does not delegate you to one of the angels who serves Him. He is always waiting on you to come to Him.

> God desires to have a meaningful relationship with you daily. With Him, you are never put on hold and you never have to stand in line.

After reading it over and over again for years, I am still blown away by the reality of this verse: "Draw near to God, and he will draw near to you" (James 4:8). This is a call for us to come near to God and pursue Him intentionally. Because of what Christ accomplished on the cross, you have the capacity to approach God. You can enter into His presence. In fact, He desires to have your love and complete allegiance to Him.

Think of it this way: *You can go to God anytime, anywhere, about anything.* Through Jesus Christ, you have direct access to God.

When we think of becoming fit, we most often think of this in relationship to the human body. We call this physical fitness. But it is rare that we think about spiritual fitness. I want to challenge you to completely adjust your mind-set about this. Why?

This book is a call to intentionally raise the level of your fitness in five pivotal areas of your life. This holistic approach becomes a winning plan. The degree of your fitness in these five areas will determine your level of impact and influence upon others.

Of these five areas, none is more important than your spiritual life and its level of fitness. Yes, I have said this twice before and this makes three times: *As your spiritual life goes, so goes the rest of your life.* If you cannot be consistent and successful in developing your spiritual life, it will negatively affect the other four areas of your fitness. Moreover, if you achieve some semblance of success in the other four areas without a healthy spiritual life, it will all be for nothing. As Jesus put it, "What does it profit a man to gain the whole world and forfeit his soul?" (Mark 8:36 ESV).

It is your spiritual life that will command into order the physical, relational, financial, and emotional areas of your life. Why do I believe this?

When the Bible speaks, God speaks. What God says, He means. Look at what God says here: "But have nothing to do with pointless and silly myths. Rather, train yourself in godliness. For the training of the body has limited benefit, but godliness is beneficial in every way, since it holds promise for the present life and also for the life to come" (1 Tim. 4:7-8). Vigorously exercise yourself in responding to God personally and passionately.

Just as an athlete trains his body and calls it into submission to his will, we need to call our spiritual life into complete submission to the will of God. This takes self-control, personal discipline, and intentional, specific actions.

Five Intentional, Specific Actions to Become Spiritually Fit

Almost daily, I see a reference to exercises that will help your belly become flat and appear slimmer than ever before. While I do not doubt the effectiveness of the exercises, I am intrigued by the appeal to take action.

Just as this is true for your physical body, it is even more true for your spiritual life. Since your spiritual life and its fitness are dependent on you taking the necessary actions—exercises, we might say—to develop it, I want to suggest five actions to take daily to help you become spiritually fit.

Action 1: Resolve: I will develop my spiritual life daily.

At some level, you have already accomplished this today. Why? You are reading this book. You are reading this chapter. You are making a voluntary choice to develop your spiritual life today.

The choices you make about your spiritual development will influence and, at times, determine the kind of choices you make in every other area of your life. Nothing happens in isolation, especially decision-making.

Therefore, each morning when you rise, say to yourself, "I will develop my spiritual life today." Your life, and all it has the potential to become, begins right here daily. It begins with a deep and disciplined resolve. This is the kind of resolve that is not determined by your personal feelings each day or the weather outside. It is determined by your personal conviction, "I must do whatever is necessary to develop my spiritual walk with God today."

Action 2: Surrender: I will release my life to God daily.

Jeana and I have seven grandchildren: Peyton, Reese, Parker, Beckham, Jack, Norah, and Maya. We have cherished every hug and kiss. One of the joys when they are just beginning to crawl and advancing to walk is when they reach their arms upward for us to pick them up. As a parent or grandparent, we would never deny them this opportunity. So what do we do? When they reach up and surrender themselves to us, we reach down, pick them up, and embrace them fully.

This is what God does for us in an even greater way when we surrender and release ourselves completely to Him. When we surrender to God, we are like children who are reaching our arms upward, hoping He will reach down and pick us up. This is a wonderful picture of a spiritual reality we should experience daily.

As you resolve to develop your spiritual life, you will learn the power of surrendering your life to God daily. Surrendering your life to God means to release your life completely to God. You become like a little child, raising your arms upward and placing yourself into the arms of God.

When you choose to do this, you are turning away from the power of your own ability and leaning completely upon the power of Christ. Any time we turn away from sinful choices and the power of trusting in our own ability, we are practicing repentance. When we have a change of mind about the way we want to live, that is repentance.

Repentance is not just an initial action in order to receive salvation in Christ alone, nor is it simply apologizing or verbally confessing a sin committed; rather, it is an ongoing action in the life of anyone who wants to walk with God intimately and passionately. Changing the way we think and how we want to live is a needed action to becoming spiritually fit. Making a decision to walk away from sin and toward God is always good. This is the power of repentance.

> Repentance is not just an initial action in order to receive salvation in Christ alone, nor is it simply apologizing or verbally confessing a sin committed; rather, it is an ongoing action in the life of anyone who wants to walk with God intimately and passionately.

Releasing your life to God involves not only repentance, but also humility. When a child gives up her own will and reaches her arms upward to you, she is practicing a strong form of humility. Surrendering to God daily always involves both repentance and humility.

Humility is the practice of making yourself low before God and others. It is the opposite of pride. While pride calls you to lean upon yourself, humility calls you to lean upon God. Practicing humility before God and others is a remarkable testimony of a life surrendered to God.

Therefore, daily surrender your life to God. In other words, determine, "I will release my life to God daily."

Action 3: I will read the Bible daily.

The Bible is God's Word. It's what God says to me, and to all people. Thus, I need to read the Bible every day.

Through the years, I have witnessed thousands of Christians who live out their faith. Almost without exception, those who read the Bible daily are set apart from the others.

Former trucking magnate J. B. Hunt used to tell me that the Bible was his road map for the way he wanted to live. Mr. Hunt used to drive trucks all over America before he and Mrs. Hunt began their company. While he lived on the road, the map of our country became important to him. It led him to his desired destination.

Mr. Hunt began his day reading the Bible. He used to tell me it would take him at least eighteen months to read through the Bible once, but he read through the entire Bible several times in his life. It was his roadmap for the way he wanted to live.

Let the life of J. B. Hunt inspire you to read the Bible daily. If an extraordinarily busy and wealthy man like Mr. Hunt knew he still needed to read the Bible and make it a priority each day of his life, hopefully it will inspire you to do the same.

This is a daily discipline that is imperative to practice in order to be fit spiritually. I promise you this: You cannot be all God wants you to be if you do not read the Bible. It is impossible.

When you read the Bible, read it seeking. As you hang on every word from the Bible, you are seeking God's will and intention for your life. You are seeking for God to speak to your life. Remember, when the Bible speaks, God speaks!

Every time you read the Bible seeking a word from God, it will alter your life and mind-set throughout the day and beyond. The Bible is what it says it is. Psalm 119:105 says, "Your word is a lamp for my feet and a light on my path." In this spiritually dark world, we need God to shine a light on how we need to live and where we need to go in life. This is only found in reading the Bible daily.

When you read the Bible, read it attempting to grow. A baby graduates from milk to meat. For us, the Bible is like our meat. It nourishes us. It helps us grow in our faith and commitment to Christ. Every genuine Christian needs to grow.

As you read the Bible seeking, your faith will grow. The Bible will mature you. The psalmist says it profoundly in Psalm 119:25: "Give me life through your word." I promise that when you read the Bible daily, God's Word will empower you with life greater than you have ever experienced before.

As you seek the Lord through reading the Bible and grow in Christ, there is one other aspect of reading the Bible I have found to be important. Read the Bible systematically.

Develop a consistency in your Bible reading. Many methods are available online or in print. Find a system that works for you and lean into doing it consistently.

I have read the Bible through at least one time each year since 1990. For several years now, I have followed a system, but within that system, I have done it in various ways. Therefore, as I write this book, I have read through the Bible no fewer than twenty-seven times since 1990. Before then, I always read consistently, but I never had a planned, intentional way to read it through completely.

I can tell you from my own life, nothing has shaped me more than reading through God's Word daily. While I do it systematically,

I do it seeking to hear God speak to me about my life and yearning to have His Word mature me.

Action 4: I will talk to God daily.

God speaks to you when you read the Bible. In response to God, talk to Him daily. We call this prayer. Prayer is a conversation with God. It involves listening to God speak to you through His Word and talking to Him about your life.

Since you can go to God anytime, anywhere, about anything that's going on in your life, choose to talk to God daily. Again, create your own system of prayer or adopt someone else's. If nothing else, make a list of things you are concerned about in your own life, your family, your church, your career and business, your future, your finances, your country, and any concerns you have for other people. Pray for them each day and look for God to walk into those situations personally and powerfully. God answers prayer!

I keep my prayer list in the Notes app on my iPad. My list changes continually as I watch God respond to my prayers. As this happens, I can easily change my list because of the simplicity of using the iPad. Again, find your way and just do it!

Action 5: I will take the necessary actions to be fit spiritually.

The title of this chapter is "Live Intentionally." This is a call to self-control, self-discipline, and intentional, specific actions. This is a time for you to take action personally.

Many people hear words like *discipline* and *intentional* and think we're talking about salvation by works. Of course, salvation by works is unbiblical, but that's not what I mean here. Salvation is by grace through faith, but faith in the Bible is always connected to a life of discipleship. There is an intimate connection between discipline and discipleship—you can see it in the two words! You are saved by God's grace, but once you are saved, you must cultivate your relationship with Him by living an intentional and disciplined life.

What kind of personal actions am I referring to? The very actions I have written about in this chapter:

- I will develop my spiritual life daily.
- I will release my life to God daily.
- I will read the Bible daily.
- I will talk to God daily.

These are intentional and necessary actions to take in order to become fit spiritually. You can do this, so begin taking these actions today. This will place you in the best position to have a successful, godly life. This is what it means to live intentionally.

SECTION 2

Living Fit Physically

CHAPTER 5

Live Fully

Periodically, I pray, "Lord, I surrender all of me to all of You so that all of You will live in and through all of me." Daily, I pray, "Lord, I surrender all of my mind, my will, my emotions, my body, my spirit, my tongue, my attitude, my motives, my past, my present, my future, my dreams, and my goals to You." These prayers and other prayers like them lead me to a full and complete surrender to the lordship of Jesus Christ.

This is the beginning point of realizing that your spiritual life is not and cannot be compartmentalized from the rest of your life. Nothing happens in isolation. It never has and it never will. Everything is connected. Therefore, live fully.

This is significant for each of us to understand. As we enter into this second section about living fit physically, we need to understand that our commitment to living fit physically is connected to our commitment to living fit spiritually. Furthermore, it is connected to every part of our life.

As we established in the first chapter of this book, when the Bible speaks, God speaks. Therefore, we need to read the Bible as God's words to us. For example, 1 Thessalonians 5:23 says, "Now may the God of peace himself sanctify you completely. And may your whole spirit, soul, and body be kept sound and blameless at the coming of our Lord Jesus Christ." Did you know that you do not have the power in and of yourself to separate yourself from sin?

Separating us from our sin is the exclusive work of God. The gospel of Jesus Christ initiates His peace as the reconciling power that sets us apart from the world. God's peace will sanctify us. This means He sets us apart, makes us holy, and purifies us for holy use. It is God's work through the person of the Holy Spirit that sets you apart completely. Then a bold statement follows that says, when interpreted accurately, God wants all of us—body, soul, and spirit—to be surrendered fully to Jesus. It says, "and may your whole spirit, soul, and body be kept sound and blameless."

I do not think the issue here is the individual parts of what we are; the issue is that God wants each of us to be committed to Him wholly and fully. In other words, His sanctifying power sets our whole, complete selves apart for holy use—not just part of us. When we think of someone we love, we do not think of just their spirit, soul, or body. We think of them as a whole person. We are whole beings.

When we begin thinking this way, it will empower us to be kept sound and blameless until the Lord returns to this earth personally and visibly. Therein lies the call in this chapter to live fully.

Three Insights to Help You Understand How to Live Fully

I want to take that which is seemingly complex and simplify it as much as possible and communicate it clearly. Here are three insights we must consider and understand if we are going to live more fully for Christ.

Insight 1: Your entire life is connected; it is not compartmentalized.

One of the most distorted ideas many people have about faith is that their faith is one part of their life, one piece of the pie. In other words, there is no convergence of one's faith in the workplace or politics or recreation or any other segment of life. This is wrong. Your spiritual life is not and cannot be compartmentalized from the rest of your life. If you see it as divided or separated from the rest of your life, you are not seeing things correctly or clearly.

This mentality creates people who see themselves as Christ-followers on Sunday, but Monday through Saturday they are following their own lead, not God's. This is a horrible testimony of the gospel of Jesus Christ. It is contradictory to the call of Jesus for each of us. As we go, we are to make disciples of all the nations.

This compartmentalized approach to Christianity is unfounded in Scripture. Never do we see faith separated from the rest of life. Your faith in Jesus Christ is a call to follow Him daily. It goes with you everywhere. You do not have the power or authority to check Jesus at the door like you check your bags in an airport. He goes with you every day, everywhere.

Therefore, refuse to see your life as being compartmentalized. You are not divided and you cannot live like you are. Every part of you is connected to the rest of you, and every part of your life is connected to the rest of your life.

> **Refuse to see your life as being compartmentalized. You are not divided and you cannot live like you are.**

When Jesus Christ is the center of your life, He impacts each and every part of it. Imagine your entire life as a circle. Right in the middle of this circle is your personal relationship with Jesus Christ. From the middle of your circle, arrows go outward toward each segment of your life.

This imaginary circle becomes an illustration of how you must see your faith and its place in your life. It impacts each segment of your life either positively or negatively, depending on how fit it is.

The implications of believing this are powerful. As your spiritual life goes, so goes the rest of your life. The more fit you are spiritually, the more fit you are likely to become physically, relationally, financially, and emotionally. If any of these areas of life are unhealthy, it will negatively affect the other areas.

When your understanding of this increases and you begin to live out your faith through each area of your life, you will begin to grasp the enormous influence that God wants your faith to have in and through your life. Therefore, the first insight to help you understand how to live fully is to realize your entire life is connected; it is not compartmentalized.

Insight 2: You are a whole person, not just parts.

It is evident from research and study that the overall main emphasis of this biblical text is not on what parts comprise the human personality. This is important to understand.

The apostle Paul was not teaching a psychology or anatomy class in an academic setting. While some may be motivated by figuring out who we are and what we are made of, Paul's goal in this text was to tell people that the God of peace, Jesus, sets every part of our humanity apart to live unto Himself wholly.

If you see yourself as being comprised only of various parts, then you will reason in your mind that the compartmentalization of your faith is acceptable and that it is separate from every other part of your life. Again, this is a mistake and an improper way to see yourself.

You are a whole person, not just the collection of the parts of your person. Romans 12:1 states, "Therefore, brothers and sisters, in view of the mercies of God, I urge you to present your bodies as a living sacrifice, holy and pleasing to God; this is your true worship." When the reference here says "present your bodies," this is a not a reference to the matter of your body only, leaving out your soul and spirit, as noted in 1 Thessalonians 5:23. This phrase, "present your bodies," is a call to each follower of Jesus Christ to surrender our entire person to live in a holy way that is pleasing to God. When we present all we are to God, we are giving Him our full and complete worship.

This Romans 12:1 passage compliments what 1 Thessalonians 5:23 states. Both of these Scriptures call us to live fully for God, even though they do so in a different way. The call to follow Jesus Christ is a call to surrender all we have and all we are to Him.

In understanding how to live fully, I have given you two insights to consider. The first insight is to realize your entire life is connected; it is not compartmentalized. The second insight is to see yourself as a whole person, not just parts of your person. With a greater understanding now of how to live fully, I want to give you the third insight that may help you further.

Insight 3: You have a spirit, soul, and body; you are not just a physical blob of human matter.

We now realize and know that this passage ultimately states that Jesus sets every segment of our human personality apart, to live unto Him wholly in order to live holy before others. It reminds us that not one part of our person eludes the sanctification process of the Holy Spirit. It is a call to you and to me to follow and live fully for God.

While the main call of 1 Thessalonians 5:23 is to give our whole selves to God, we cannot contradict the words it uses to do so. As the verse says, you have a spirit, soul, and body. This is undeniable. While interpretation of this does vary, it does not negate what Scripture says. I think this is very important to recognize in our culture today. Why do I believe this?

Presently, the sanctity and dignity of human life is being greatly devalued. If we dumb down the uniqueness and the intricate details about the reality of the human creation God made, we will also dumb down the sanctity and dignity of human life. If we see ourselves or other people as simply a piece of human matter—a clump of cells—that is here today and gone tomorrow, we will not recognize the realities of eternity or human dignity. We will not recognize how God has given each of us a purpose in life that is both meaningful and valuable.

You are not just a physical blob of human matter. You have been created by God in His image. You have been wonderfully made.

While each of us is a "whole person," we are also comprised of various parts that have been designed with purpose. We cannot just refer to Romans 12:1 as I have mentioned and explained earlier in this chapter, but we also must look at Romans 12:2, because it helps us understand more clearly the undeniable reality mentioned in 1 Thessalonians 5:23.

Romans 12:2 says, "Do not be conformed to this age, but be transformed by the renewing of your mind, so that you may discern what is the good, pleasing, and perfect will of God." Transformation and change occur in a progressive manner by the renewing of the mind. As your mind, the way you think, and your mind-set becomes more like Christ, you will be more able to discern what is the good, pleasing, and perfect will of God. There is a definite recognition that even though you are a whole person, your whole person becomes more of what God wants you to be when your mind is being renewed and is being transformed the way you think and live out God's Word.

Considering all I have stated in this chapter about these verses, I do believe we have a spirit. First Corinthians 6:17 says, "But anyone joined to the Lord is one spirit with him." I believe when we come to Christ in salvation, our spirit unites with the Holy Spirit.

First Thessalonians 5:23 states that you have a soul. Each person has a mind, a will, and emotions. Could these represent the soul? Or, said another way, is the soul comprised of the mind, the will, and emotions? Only God knows the answer to this. Yet, if there is anything that needs to be sanctified and set apart to God only, it is the mind, the will, and the emotion. Left on their own, they are dangerous and destructive to your life.

First Thessalonians 5:23 also says you have a body. While the body decays, it also needs to be sanctified and fully set apart to honor God.

I believe each of us has four major problems in life. We have a mind problem, a will problem, an emotion problem, and a body problem. Any of these four problems, individually, could have a major impact on your life. If you lose control of all four of these problems at one time, the impact could destroy your life.

This is where sanctification becomes your hope while you are living out your faith on this earth. At salvation, your spirit is united with the Holy Spirit and is now permitted to work in and through your entire life. God's sanctifying process in you brings your mind, will, emotion and body into submission to God.

> We have a mind problem, a will problem, an emotional problem, and a body problem.

Yes, your entire life is connected; it is not compartmentalized. Please see yourself as a whole person, not just a collection of parts. God has created you uniquely and wonderfully, full of intricate details. As 1 Thessalonians 5:23 states, you have a spirit, soul, and body.

For Clarity

While interpretations of certain parts of 1 Thessalonians 5:23 will vary, I want to make sure I am very clear. As I have stated throughout this chapter, I believe God's ultimate intention is for our entire being, the whole person, to be set apart to live only for God.

Who I am as a creation and what I am comprised of as a human being will remain mysterious on this side of heaven. But it is not a mystery to me that God is calling me and He is calling you to live fully for Him.

CHAPTER 6

Live Orderly

While God determines your number of days on this earth, you will determine the quality and effectiveness of each of these days. The healthier you are spiritually, physically, relationally, financially, and emotionally, the greater the impact you will have each day you are on this earth.

The more fit you are spiritually, the more fit you should attempt to be physically. Health and wellness do not begin physically, but spiritually. While most people have never connected these two, the Christian cannot separate them from one another. When you follow Christ personally—as we discussed in the previous chapter—spirit, soul, and body are to be set apart for God and His glory.

For Christ to be in control of your life means He is also in control of your body. Ordering your body into submission to God takes personal discipline as well as divine intervention. This does not happen easily or naturally, but it does need to happen.

An Inside Story

Everyone has a story. I want to tell you mine.

Athletics played a major role in the younger years of my life. Growing up in Texas, it was all about Friday night lights in Texas high school football. I loved every minute of it.

While eating healthy was not much on the agenda during that time, working out and taking care of my body was important even then. The hot August sun of south central Texas and the grueling experience of two-a-day workouts in full uniform for at least two weeks prior to the beginning of school ignited me.

I loved the game of football so much that I wanted to be a coach. I had a personal vision of coaching football one day in high school, college, and then in the pros. To this very day, I still love the game in every way and would still love to coach at every level.

But when God redirected my life, vision, and passion, He also redirected my future.

Earning my college degree, followed by graduating with my master's and doctorate degrees, led to an excessively busy life. Simultaneously, marriage and family, as well as pastoring churches while earning my degrees, left little to no time in my mind to pay much attention to myself physically.

While I was earning my doctoral degree and pastoring a church full-time, I let myself go physically. My weight was out of control and it affected me in every way.

When I finished college and stopped competing on a football field, I hung physical fitness up completely. I lost all motivation for taking better care of myself and convinced myself there was no time for it.

It was not until completing my doctoral degree and focusing on pastoring a church that I determined I needed to take more control of myself not just spiritually, but physically. The growing demands of my job and, by God's grace, my increased maturity in life, moved me into a new day of taking better care of my body.

I began to connect the dots between my spiritual life and physical life. I stopped seeing them as separate and realized they were united in who I was as a person. This has been a continual growing process for me. I assume it probably is for most people.

Today, working out six days a week is pretty normal for me. Even with my crazy schedule of leading a large multi-campus church, speaking around the country, writing articles and books, and serving in various ways regionally or nationally, there are two strong personal commitments I have in my life.

I believe these commitments have advanced my development as a person. The first thing I do each day of my life is spend time with God, prioritizing my personal walk with Him and development in Him and His Word. This is absolutely non-negotiable, and has been a personal practice for decades, regardless of travel. This sixty to ninety-minute time with God has transformed my life. There is no way I can navigate to being healthy spiritually without this daily time with God.

Additionally, usually six mornings a week, I give an hour to physical fitness. I jog most of these six days, and two days a week I combine my running with strength and conditioning training. While exercising, I listen to podcasts on leadership and professional equipping, as well as the teaching of God's Word by others. Joining the physical and spiritual helps me not only justify the time, but redeem the time to grow spiritually and professionally.

These two disciplines have added both quality and effectiveness to my days for many years. By God's grace alone, I pray I will be able to do the same in decades to come.

This is my story. What's yours?

Ordering Your Life with Discipline

Discipline is doing the right thing even when we do not want to. Living a disciplined life—even related to physical fitness—is imperative to living an orderly life.

After several decades of rising early each morning to begin my day with God, it is still not easy. Even after working out for decades and understanding the value of it in my life, it is still not easy for me to do. This is why I bring order to my life with discipline.

First Timothy 4:7-8 says, "But have nothing to do with pointless and silly myths. Rather, train yourself in godliness. For the training of the body has limited benefit, but godliness is beneficial in every way, since it holds promise for the present life and also for the life to come." The Scripture instructs us here to disregard false teachings and pointless ideologies that are unfit for followers of Christ. Rather, you and I are called upon to train ourselves in godliness.

The word *train* means to exercise like an athlete would for an athletic performance or competition. The kind of discipline, rigor, and sacrifice that an athlete exerts as he trains is the same kind of discipline, rigor, and sacrifice you should have in your spiritual life. As committed as an athlete is to his training, you should be even more committed to training yourself in godliness. What does this take? It takes self-discipline, self-control, and self-sacrifice.

> As committed as an athlete is to his training, you should be even more committed to training yourself in godliness.

The Bible tells us that the training of the body has limited benefit, since it does not last forever. Conversely, rigorous commitment to walking with God will result in godly living and thinking. This rigor to godliness is advantageous in every way because it does not just direct our life while on this earth, but it also prepares us for life eternally.

I know some people may use this passage in 1 Timothy to excuse themselves from taking care of their physical bodies. To some, it may appear that Christians are exempt from physical exertion. But this Scripture does not say that exercise has zero benefit, but that its benefit is limited, since it is only beneficial on this earth. Therefore, we are not excused to live as we desire. The Holy Spirit sets us apart to pursue holiness and to live with self-control.

When I began to use technology to pour biblical teaching and spiritual equipping into my time of physical fitness, it really increased the quality of my workouts. Before then, I struggled some with justifying the time. I do know the Scripture tells us that while there are benefits to both physical and spiritual training, it is spiritual fitness and its benefits that last for an eternity. So, both spiritual and physical fitness are important, but not equally important. This wise and right perspective is very important for each of us to have. Again, while God determines your number of days on this earth, you will determine the quality and effectiveness of each of these days. I believe you do this with a commitment to being both spiritually and physically fit.

Ordering your life with discipline is so important to your future. It really takes self-discipline to bring order to your life. How disciplined are you?

Self-Discipline Leads to Order

A lack of self-discipline will usually lead to a life of disorder. I believe it is important to understand that God is a God of order, not disorder.

As Creator of the heavens and the earth, God created everything and everyone with order. He did not do anything flippantly. Everything and everyone was created with order and purpose. All the structures God created were made to bring Him glory and provide a sense of order for everyone and everything in the world. From creation to family, from government to church, each was created with order and to bring order into the world today.

In the New Testament church, God elevated order. When the apostle Paul was writing to the church in Corinth, he called them to order and unity in the operation of their spiritual gifts in the church. Not wanting them to abuse their spiritual gifts, which would result in chaos and disorder, he boldly called them to operate in worship in an orderly manner. We can learn something about God and the principle of orderliness from 1 Corinthians 14.

In 1 Corinthians 14:33 we read, "Since God is not a God of disorder but of peace." Then in 1 Corinthians 14:40, Paul gives a strong call when he writes, "But everything is to be done decently and in order." From these two verses, we learn the principle of orderliness. Contextually, this principle is in reference to the church operating with one another and in public meetings for worship. While this is the original context in 1 Corinthians, we know that because God is a God of order and because He is unchanging, God's orderliness can be applied to all of life.

Sin causes chaos, not God. Sin causes disorder, not God. I believe not only that God is a God of order and has put in place systems and structures to create order in our relationships, but He also wants us to live orderly.

Living with self-control is a fruit of the Holy Spirit. As He is filling us with His Spirit and we are walking in step with His Spirit, we will live with self-control. This creates order in our personal lives.

Therefore, self-discipline leads to order. Ordering your body into submission to God takes personal discipline as well as divine intervention. Without God and the power of His Spirit, we will live runaway, chaotic, and disorderly lives.

As I mentioned earlier, Romans 12:2 is a call to present our bodies as a living sacrifice to God that is holy and pleasing to Him.

Giving your body to God is giving your all to God. God wants even your body to glorify Him. This will not happen without self-discipline that leads to order.

Your Body Matters to God

Your body matters to God because He created you. Disregarding the value of your body as a human being does not take away from the value God intends for it to have in your life.

Self-worship is never God's intent for any of us. We are here to worship Him and extend His glory to every corner of this universe. I'm not in any way saying we should worship the human body, but that disciplining it is a way of worshipping God. A healthy understanding and a balanced biblical view about your physical body will help give you the right perspective.

Each of us recognizes, to some level, the value of the body. If we did not, we would never take a shower, look in the mirror, go into clothing stores, or go to the doctor. But we do each of these and more because we do place some value on the human body.

Your body matters to God. In I Corinthians 6:19-20, God says to us, "Don't you know that your body is a temple of the Holy Spirit who is in you, whom you have from God? You are not your own, for you were bought with a price. So glorify God with your body." If you are a genuine follower of Jesus Christ, your body is the temple or sanctuary of God. Your body is where the Holy Spirit lives and dwells. Yes, your body matters to God.

But your body also belongs to God. When you acknowledged Christ and His sacrificial and substitutionary death for you and determined to receive the cleansing power of His blood that removed all your sin, you submitted to God's ownership of your body. It does not exist for you, but for Him. It is not here to satisfy your desires, but to glorify God.

Any abuse of our bodies with food, harm, or personal sin not only disrupts and disorders, but can even destroy our bodies. The moment we come to Christ, the human body and everything else becomes the Lord's. It all belongs to Him. Therefore, the body in which the Holy Spirit dwells should always bring the greatest glory to God possible. Your body matters to God.

You Can Do Something

I could die at any time on any day. So could you. Even with my disciplined commitment to being fit not just spiritually, but also physically, I am one breath away from eternity.

I decided many years ago that I want to operate at maximum capacity as long as I am physically able. I determined to do something about it—not for the sake of performance, but for the sake of the cause.

Jesus Christ is my cause. I want my walk with Him to be vibrant. I want my ministry to His Church to be effective. I want my leadership for the future to be inspired. I want my commitment to His Great Commission—the commandment Jesus gave to the Church to make disciples of all nations—to be focused.

These things cannot and will not happen without self-discipline, self-control, and personal order. Therefore, I concluded for God to be in control of my life meant that He also needed to be in control of my body. As much as possible with all my limitations, I want to live an orderly life.

I determined to do something about it. Will you? Determine to give order a new place in your life. Start wherever you are right now. Find your level. Go forward.

You can do something.

CHAPTER 7

Live Reasonably

Cultural deceptions are dangerous and destructive. In this age of fake news, truth seems to be minimized and even lost. As these realities converge, they have created unrealistic expectations about many things. This taints our judgment and discernment, leading us to operate our lives in an unreasonable manner that, at times, can become irrational.

Jeremiah 9:6 states these frightening words, "You live in a world of deception." Sadly, this did not just occur in Jeremiah's day, but is happening now. Even among friends, Jeremiah warned, "No one tells the truth. They have taught their tongues to speak lies" (Jer. 9:5). These are tragic statements about the power of deception.

Deception misleads. Deception maligns. Deception lies.

As it was in the day of Jeremiah, it is today. We live in a day of deception. The greatest deceptions being communicated in our culture today are deceptions relating to the human body. Let me explain why I believe this.

Manipulative marketing via television, web, and print media lead us to think we can look like some man or woman whose image has been airbrushed. Airbrushing manipulates a photo through a process of editing that removes the imperfections of the human body. In this digital age, if a person can communicate in any way technologically, they can easily learn to edit photos and make someone appear to be something that, in reality, that person is not.

Manipulative marketing lures you into becoming unreasonable with your expectations and irrational in your judgment. After seeing something time and time again with your eyes, it appears to your subconscious as truth. This is dangerous and can be destructive.

For example, how many miracle-working beauty products do you see and hear about through some form of media? You are led to believe that when you purchase this product and apply it to your skin, in just a few days you will look twenty years younger. Now, I would love to look twenty years younger. Who wouldn't? I think just about anyone who is forty years of age or older would love to look twenty years younger!

I am not stating miracle-working beauty products never live up to any of their promises. Perhaps they do. But what is concerning is the vision created in the minds of people that is just not reality.

Another example of manipulative marketing is the promotion of a pill or a process that will produce magical weight loss. In fact, you can eat whatever you want and as much of it as you want, and experience this magic weight loss. This sounds so appealing! Then before your eyes, before and after photos fly across the screen, encouraging you to believe this is all really possible.

But is it possible? Eat all you want and whatever you want, take this pill or do this exercise for just five minutes a day, and look what will happen! You can experience miraculous weight loss!

I can assure you as a person who must be continually conscious of his weight, this is not the way it works. In fact, from a recent study published in the *New England Journal of Medicine*, we know that 30 percent of the world's population is affected by weight problems, with 10 percent being classified as obese.[1] A good portion of our world's population struggles with this issue.

If I ate whatever I wanted and as much as I wanted, I would continually feel very sluggish. If I compounded that practice by never exercising, not only would I feel sluggish and slow, but my weight would easily get out of control.

These things are just not reasonable. You cannot create unreasonable goals and expectations regarding your physical fitness.

The subtitle of this book needs to resonate with you as you work through this content: *Make Your Life Count by Pursuing a Healthy You.*

Health is a journey. Health is a process. Journeys and processes take time. Therefore, as you set your sail to your desired destination, make sure your destination is reasonable. If it is not, you may end up in a place in your life that is nowhere close to where you really want to be.

> **Health is a journey. Health is a process. Journeys and processes take time.**

Should we be concerned with our looks or with our health? Health is much more comprehensive than just the way we look. If appearance is your only goal, you will probably live disappointed most of the time. Conversely, if health and wellness are your goals, then you will increase your potential to achieve these with self-control, self-discipline, and focus.

My appeal to you in this section and in this chapter more specifically is to live reasonably. As you are on your way to living fit physically, live reasonably. How do you do this?

Three Ways to Live Reasonably in This Day of Unreason

I want to share three ways you can live reasonably, even in this day of unreason. As irrationality occurs relating to the human body, how do we persevere and live reasonably?

1. You are created in the image of God.

Genesis 1:27 states these powerful words, "So God created man in his own image; he created him in the image of God; he created them male and female." Only God created male and female. This first reference here to the term *man* refers to all humanity—not just male, but also female.

Scholars have debated for years what the image of God truly means. Human creation is given the capacity to reason. Human creation is given the entrustment of stewarding all God has created. Human creation is given a mind, a will, and emotions. We are the most unique and crowning creation of God, the only beings made in His image. We are not animals, and animals are not humans. Before the fall recorded in Genesis 3, we were without sin.

Interestingly, it is mentioned that God has created both male and female. These are two distinct genders made in the image of God. Their unique distinctiveness is a prized creation of God. God created male and female uniquely, designing each so they could come together physically in order to be fruitful, multiply, and fill the earth. Regardless of what our deceptive culture promotes in this day of unreason, gender is not fluid.

So in this day of unreason, you can live reasonably when you always have first and foremost in your mind and heart: *I have been created in the image of God.* As His image bearers, our attributes are unique among all of His creation, resulting in us being special in His eyes. Once God made us as the crowning glory of His creation, Genesis 1:31 tells us, "God saw all that he had made, and it was very good indeed."

Keep perspective in this day of unreason. Live reasonably by knowing you are made in the image of God.

2. There is no one else like you.

While each of us as human beings are made in the image of God, each of us is created uniquely by God. This uniqueness is real and should be celebrated. There is no one else like you.

Science affirms our uniqueness because it declares that while some people may have a similar DNA, no two people have the exact same DNA. Identical twins are as close as possible, but even then, medical science does not believe they have the exact same DNA. Again, there is no one else like you.

This is declared with precision in Psalm 139:13-16. It states,

For it was you who created my inward parts; you knit me together in my mother's womb. I will praise you because I have been remarkably and wondrously made. Your works are wondrous, and I know this very well. My bones were not hidden from you when I was made in secret, when I was formed in the depths of the earth. Your eyes saw me when I was formless; all my days were written in your book and planned before a single one of them began.

What a powerful illustration of how God created us. There is no one else like you.

With precision, exactness, and conciseness, God meticulously made you. He put you together while you were in your mother's womb. He did not make one mistake with you.

You are special. Each member of your family is special. Each friend is special. Your boss is special. Each employee is special. Your spouse is special. The person you struggle with relationally is special, even as special as you are.

Our God has made you meticulously. Do not miss this: There is no one else like you.

God has made you powerfully. As one of His created human beings, your creation testifies to the majesty, power, and glory of God. David praised God when he thought about how he was made so remarkably by God. In awe, he marveled at how God had made him so extraordinarily and powerfully.

We take our creation and the birth of children so much for granted; we have forgotten each stage and moment is miraculous! It is miraculous that we are even born, that we are even brought to life. We should always—and I mean always—give God praise for making us so wondrously.

God has made you knowingly. He has known everything about you from your beginning and all the way until your end. God is sovereign over your life and over your death. He was never surprised and never will be.

In this day of unreason, it will help you to live reasonably when you reflect upon and even celebrate how God has made you so meticulously and miraculously. There is no one like you.

How do you make sense in this day of unreason? Never forget these realities that initiate the action and direction for your life: You are created in the image of God, and there is no one else like you.

3. You are destined with purpose.

In chapter 3, I went into greater detail about purpose. I encouraged you to declare:

- I believe God has a purpose for my life.
- I will pursue God's purpose for my life.
- I believe nothing can hinder God's purpose for my life.
- I will serve God's purpose in my generation.

These things are true and need to be declared by each of us. In relationship to our creation, I also want to declare today: *You are destined with purpose.*

The prophet Jeremiah was able to keep his balance in an age of unreason because of what he writes in the first chapter of his book. Jeremiah 1:4-5 says, "The word of the LORD came to me: I chose you before I formed you in the womb; I set you apart before you were born. I appointed you a prophet to the nations." Furthermore, he writes in Jeremiah 1:10, "See, I have appointed you today over nations and kingdoms to uproot and tear down, to destroy and demolish, to build and plant." These two Scriptures are so very strong regarding Jeremiah's purpose.

You are also destined with purpose! Think about how purposeful God was in His creation of Jeremiah. God chose him because He knew Jeremiah so intricately in creation. Even while in his mother's womb, Jeremiah said that God destined him to be a prophet to the nations. He said Jeremiah would have a strong influence on nations and kingdoms.

Think about the power of all this. Jeremiah was destined with purpose from the moment he was in the womb of his mother. So are you! You are destined with purpose! While mystery may exist about what your purpose may be, you can know for certain it is significant.

Please understand that the only way you can live reasonably in this day of unreason is by remembering:

- You are made in the image of God.
- There is no one else like you.
- You are destined with purpose.

This becomes an enormous tension as you live in and navigate the quagmire of so much cultural deception.

Living fit physically is not easy to achieve. This is why you need divine intervention in your life. Your spiritual fitness *does* and *should* influence your physical fitness.

> **Living fit physically is not easy to achieve. This is why you need divine intervention in your life.**

Our flesh is so powerful and our culture is so deceptive. I really believe you need divine intervention in an ongoing manner in order to pursue a healthy you.

Keep These Thoughts in Your Heart

Just as we do not have the same spiritual gifts, we do not have the same physical bodies. We are created uniquely, meticulously, powerfully, and knowingly. This journey to health is not about looking like another person physically.

Being fit physically always takes into account your body's uniqueness as God has created you; therefore, you cannot have unreasonable goals and expectations for your fitness. Accepting your uniqueness as God's creation will lead you to live reasonably, not unrealistically.

You are created in the image of God. There is no one else like you. You are destined with purpose.

CHAPTER 8

Live Knowingly

God wants you to live fit physically, not just spiritually. Our commitment to living fit physically is connected to our commitment to living fit spiritually. The connection between these two is undeniable. Remember, your spiritual life is connected to every other part of your life.

Most devout Christians have specific convictions that certain things are just wrong. In their belief system, most hold some level of moral conviction, even though they may not adhere to some of their personal convictions as faithfully as they once did.

What I have found interesting through the years is that few Christians take their physical fitness as seriously as their spiritual fitness. In fact, most do not even have personal health and wellness on their radar. They do not see or recognize that God is concerned about how we care for the body He has entrusted to each of us.

As I think about this and work through this delicate subject, I think many followers of Christ have this kind of perspective:

- I know I cannot justify drunkenness.
- I know I cannot justify sexual immorality.

- I know I cannot justify gossiping.
- I know I cannot justify laziness.
- I know I cannot justify divorce.

But one thing I can do is eat as much as I want and whatever I want. Therefore, we give ourselves permission.

Let me be honest with you. I have felt this way in my life. There are so many things I know are not right that I have justified in my mind at times or in seasons. We have to eat, so let's roll! Let's eat! Let's enjoy!

Eating with a friend, a family member, or even an acquaintance is an experience that deepens relationships and enriches community. This is positive and enjoyable. It should be! Sharing a table with someone is special and meaningful.

Yet, we need to know ourselves well enough that we practice self-control and self-discipline in what we eat. This is so important not only in regard to the amount of food, but also in the kind of food we consume. For example, I am a snacker. I love to go to the pantry, wander through, grab an item or two . . . or three . . . and consume them. There are many days I would rather do this than have something healthy and more substantial. If there were no such thing as chips, cookies, sweets, ice cream, and chocolate, I could eat healthy foods easily and faithfully.

I know myself very well. Therefore, I walk through many seasons in a year when I really pull back from certain kinds of food in order to eat healthy. I live knowing my own weaknesses and try to surround myself with less or no temptation regarding food.

One thing I have learned through fasting is that restraining myself is good. In fact, it deepens my commitment to live better and eat healthy when I finish the fast.

While writing this book, I have practiced a zero-sugar diet. Why would I do this? There are several reasons, but I felt like I needed to put some kind of action into my life that called me to an awareness of ongoing physical fitness.

The next time you feel you are out of control with your eating habits, do not think you will gain control by easing into it, but understand a break needs to happen in your present pattern of eating. Establish a future pattern to be pursued, at least for the next season of your life. Only you know where you are and where you need to be in your life.

While others may encourage and motivate you in your fitness, in eating, health, and physical exercise, ultimately it will be up to you. No one else has the power to determine what you do about where you are.

Feeling guilty does not result in change. Being ashamed does not result in change. Only you can make a lifestyle change in relationship to your physical fitness. Oftentimes, following a medical procedure or challenge someone has experienced, their doctor will encourage them to change their lifestyle. Fear motivates them for a while, but ultimately many return to the way things were in their previous status. Eventually, it all catches up to them, leading to an immobilized life or seeing their life decline faster than they imagined, and possibly

> No one else has the power to determine what you do about where you are.

end sooner than expected. There is something about the human persona that convinces us that we are exempt from certain things and will not pay the consequences. This is just not true.

We reap what we sow. We become what we eat. If we do not even consider a daily walk around the block, we will live to regret our lack of physical activity.

A sedentary life will lead to struggles with weight. This is happening today to children, the elderly, and everyone in between. Our challenges in American healthcare are caused by several things, but, let's not underestimate how a sedentary lifestyle has contributed to our culture's weight problems.

Any time I have lived out of control with eating and my weight, I did not like living, feeling, or looking the way I did. Thousands of people I have met through the years who have experienced some of the same issues would agree with my assessment and have felt the same way. But herein lies the problem: *We each must take action and personally own the need to make a change that will improve our physical fitness.*

For me, it took finally understanding that any lack of physical fitness linked to eating and exercise is a spiritual issue. God wants me to live and operate my life with self-control. This fruit of the Holy Spirit is needed continually in my life. For me—and I am only speaking for me—I see it all as a spiritual issue.

I know that if I see it as a spiritual issue, I will call upon God in prayer and He will empower me to work through it and lead me toward a healthy solution. For me personally, exercise itself is such a mental cleansing. My greatest struggle is mostly in regard to eating moderately and wisely.

How well do you know yourself and your practices? I want to encourage you to live knowingly.

No One Knows Your Body More Than You, So Listen to Your Body

In 1990, at a very young age, my wife, Jeana, was diagnosed with cancer. Through surgery, radiation, extreme chemotherapy, and prayer, God healed Jeana. With two very young boys, this jolted our lives in a major way.

During this experience and the years following, Jeana provided counsel and encouragement to many people located all over America who were dealing with cancer. I heard her say so many times to others what she learned through her own challenging experience. She stated, *"No one knows your body more than you, so listen to your body."*

This is not just important for those who are going through physical illness and treatment. This is also true for each of us, whether we are committed to living fit physically or not. But in all reality, it is even more true for those who are focusing on a proper commitment to physical fitness. Be wise and be reasonable. As you exercise and commit to fitness, live knowingly.

Four Specific Actions to Live Fit Physically

As we move toward concluding this section on living fit physically, I believe it is important to have some specific actions that will help you achieve your goals in relation to living fit.

These actions must come from a biblical authority so you can move forward with confidence. The Bible states in 1 Corinthians 6:19-20, "Don't you know that your body is a temple of the Holy Spirit who is in you, whom you have from God? You are not your own, for you were bought at a price. So glorify God with your body." While I have mentioned this text in a previous chapter, I want to use it now to inspire you to take action. As you are pursuing a healthy you, please consider taking these specific actions daily.

Action 1: Submit yourself to God.

There is no way you can navigate to a healthy you without submitting yourself to God daily. What should move you to do this? The Scripture teaches us in 1 Corinthians 6:19-20 that your body is the sanctuary, the temple, where God lives in you. The moment you received Christ as Savior and Lord, the Holy Spirit of God came to live inside of you. This Scripture also teaches that God has given you your body, and that Jesus redeemed your body. He knows all about you and your body because He created you uniquely and wonderfully. Therefore, you are not your own. You do not belong to yourself.

Therefore, submit yourself to God daily. If you know Christ, God lives in you, and your body is a gift to you from God. Since you do not belong to yourself anyway, you really have no other alternative except to submit yourself to God daily. Give your all to Jesus each day.

On days you exercise physically or practice eating healthy, I would encourage you to pause a moment before you begin and submit yourself to God. Ask God for self-control and self-discipline. Call upon His name and power to see you through. Never shy away from calling out to the Lord in prayer.

A worthy prayer is, *"Lord, I surrender all of me to all of You so that all of You will live in and through all of me."* Submit yourself to God humbly and daily.

Action 2: Set your body apart to God alone.

Since your body is not your own because God dwells within you, you need to live being sanctified, setting your body apart to God alone. In the earlier verses of 1 Corinthians 6, the Scripture commands us to flee sexual immorality. This is part of being set apart to God. There are some things you must flee from and some things you must run to as you submit your body to God.

Choose to live holy as you strive for holistic fitness, both spiritually and physically. Set your body apart to God alone.

Action 3: Glorify God with your body.

First Corinthians 6:20 calls us to glorify God with our bodies. Think about the various ways this is translated and interpreted.

- "So glorify God with your body." (CSB)

- "So let people see God in and through your body." (*The Message*)
- "Therefore glorify God in your body, and in your spirit, which are God's." (KJV)
- "Therefore glorify God in your body." (NASB)
- "So you must honor God with your body." (NLT)

While each of these calls upon you to glorify God with your body, each uses somewhat different language. Some are paraphrases and some are translations, but there is something to learn from this exercise.

Due to the high price paid for sin, you are called upon by God to honor Him with your body. This brings Him glory! There is one translation, the King James Version, that connects the spiritual and physical, calling upon you to glorify God in your body and in your spirit, which each belongs to God! As we do this, people can see God in and through our bodies.

> While our bodies come in all shapes and sizes, uniquely and meticulously created through the power of God, each of us is called upon to give God glory through our bodies.

While our bodies come in all shapes and sizes, uniquely and meticulously created through the power of God, each of us is called upon to give God glory through our bodies. Therefore, we need to take the necessary actions to do this in life both spiritually and physically.

Action 4: Start right now, wherever you are.

Wherever you are with your physical fitness in both exercise and eating, start right now. You cannot push rewind, wishing you had lived differently. It is too late to go backward, but not too late to go forward. Start right now wherever you are.

Be wise. Be knowledgeable. Be decisive. Chart an immediate and reasonable future. Take action.

If you want to be healthy in your forties, it begins in your late twenties and through your thirties. If you want to be healthy in your sixties, it begins in your late thirties and through your forties and fifties. For those who may be at the top end or beyond these ages, know that you can still do something about your physical fitness, even if you are just beginning.

Just begin. Do something. Take action. Start wherever you are right now.

Remember, your spiritual fitness influences your physical fitness. Moreover, when I see my fitness physically through the lens of my spiritual commitment to Christ, it provides for me the necessary motivation to be consistent, effective, and faithful. I believe that God wants each of us to be as physically fit as possible, wherever we are and at whatever level we are.

We've learned in this section on living fit physically that each of us must:

- Live fully.
- Live orderly.
- Live reasonably.
- Live knowingly.

As you are navigating to a healthy you through being fit physically, always remember these important words and worthy action: *Start right now wherever you are!*

SECTION 3

Living Fit Relationally

CHAPTER 9

Live Selflessly

As your spiritual life goes, so goes the rest of your life. Your spiritual life impacts absolutely every segment of your life. As we just learned in the previous four chapters, your spiritual life even impacts an area of life that is rarely talked about from a biblical perspective, *living fit physically.* It is time now to enter the minefield of one of the most combustible areas in life and culture today, *living fit relationally.*

In the next four chapters, we will learn about how to live fit relationally. In order to accomplish this goal, these chapters will challenge us to:

- Live selflessly
- Live lovingly
- Live connecting
- Live serving

I am not an authority in these areas and I am not sure who would say they are. If they did, I would probably question their credentials. Relationships are so important in life, and I believe we always learn new things in and through every relationship we have.

It seems that dysfunctional is the word we hear used most often regarding relationships. When one states that they are in a dysfunctional relationship, they mean that the relationship does not function effectively. Dysfunction indicates the relationship is abnormal or difficult, making it unhealthy in function.[1]

Conversely, to operate in a functional relationship means the relationship is fit, ready for service, and healthy. Being a contributing member of healthy relationships should be the goal for each of us. A functional relationship is refreshing and replenishing. A dysfunctional relationship is exasperating and exhausting. Which do you prefer, dysfunctional or functional? The health of your relationships is, in large part, a choice. What kind of relationships do you want to have in your life?

> A functional relationship is refreshing and replenishing. A dysfunctional relationship is exasperating and exhausting. Which do you prefer?

- Refreshing or exasperating?
- Replenishing or exhausting?
- Simple or complex?
- Peaceful or stressful?
- Calming or dramatic?

As a contributing member of all your relationships, you will determine which of these you want to characterize your relationships. The choice is yours.

It is undeniable that dysfunctional relationships abound in the family, the church, the workplace, the government, and in all parts of life. This present state of relationships is certainly not the will of God, but it is the current reality in our age, and, because of sin, in every age.

Oftentimes, leaders desire to talk with me about possible transitions related to their job and career status. After having conversations like these for years, I have seen a major shift within the last decade regarding what people desire in their workplace. It is interesting to me that the same thing is desired by each of these people, regardless of their level of responsibility.

While money does matter and influences the conversation to a degree, it has its limit. People will walk away from more money in order to become part of a workplace environment that is healthier than the one they are a part of presently. Furthermore, if their family is happy living here and they can find a healthier place to work, I have seen people walk away from more money and status to be a part of a functional environment at home and at work.

What does this tell us? People want to be part of a refreshing, replenishing, simple, peaceful, and calming environment. Living life is stressful enough. No one desires to have any more drama added to their life and family. At times, this may mean the family member who earns the providing income may need to practice unselfishness.

This serves as a great segue to the challenge we are now considering in this chapter about living fit relationally.

Selfishness may be one of the largest distractors in relationships. Selfishness creates dysfunction. Satisfying self in relationships consistently creates a major tidal wave of dysfunction. Selfishness is natural and normal, but it creates dysfunction and, at times, destruction in relationships.

The Mount Everest challenge before each of us relationally is to live selflessly.

> **The Mount Everest challenge before each of us relationally is to live selflessly.**

Let's Rewind

When God created the first human being, Adam, He created him for fellowship. When we go back to Genesis 1–2, God talked to Adam. Because Adam was made in the image of God, he was able to have a relationship with God where communication could occur and fellowship was experienced. Adam lived in a world where his fellowship with God was perfect.

God created us to love Him, fellowship with Him, and give Him glory. Fellowship with God is absolutely imperative for fellowship with others.

God created the first woman, Eve, to be Adam's helpmate, and they were to experience intimate fellowship. God also declared they were entrusted with the stewardship of everything in this world and told them to be fruitful and multiply, filling the earth.

When God saw all that He had made in creation, Genesis 1:31 says, "God saw all that he had made, and it was very good indeed. Evening came and then morning: the sixth day." God said clearly, "it was very good indeed." Then in Genesis 2:18 we read, "Then the LORD God said, 'It is not good for the man to be alone. I will make a helper corresponding to him.'" While God created Adam and Eve for fellowship with Him, He also created them for fellowship with one another. God made this very clear by directly saying He was going to create Eve because it was not good for Adam to be alone. Therefore, God created Eve not just for His own personal fellowship with her, but so she and Adam could have a relationship with one another.

Before sin entered the world, fellowship was perfect and meaningful. But when sin entered the world due to Adam and Eve's disobedience to God and their personal selfishness, everything changed. When Adam and Eve heard God walking in the garden, they hid from Him. They withdrew from the Lord due to their sin and shame. Their relationship with God had now changed and fellowship was impaired.

Why did this happen? Genesis 3:6 says, "The woman saw that the tree was good for food and delightful to look at, and that it was desirable for obtaining wisdom. So she took some of its fruit and ate it; she also gave some to her husband, who was with her, and he ate it." Why was this an issue? Let's let the Bible answer this question.

Earlier, as recorded in Genesis 2:16-17, we read, "And the LORD God commanded the man, 'You are free to eat from any tree of the garden, but you must not eat from the tree of the knowledge of good and evil, for on the day you eat from it, you will certainly die.'" Adam and Eve disobeyed God because they wanted to satisfy their own selfish desires by eating from the only tree they were instructed not to partake of while they were in the garden.

God created them for fellowship, and now the entire human race would be affected by this catastrophic choice of selfishness. This is one of the decisive moments in world history: sin entered the world, and our relationships with God and one another were broken.

Each of us are sinners by our nature and sinners by our choices. Thank God for His love, which He revealed in the selfless giving of His own Son, Jesus Christ, to come to the earth and die for our sin. Jesus satisfied the penalty of eternal death for all sin by becoming our substitute on the cross. First Corinthians 1:9 gives us insight into why God created us. It says, "God is faithful; you were called by him into fellowship with his Son, Jesus Christ our Lord." Through all that Jesus did for us through His bodily death and resurrection, He has called us back to our original intention and purpose of having fellowship with God, bringing glory to Him forever.

The goal of our creation was to have a personal relationship with God, but that relationship was broken by sin. Now, through the new creation Jesus began on the cross, we have the privilege of experiencing that personal relationship with God, so we can have ongoing fellowship with Him.

Selfishly versus Selflessly

Anytime we live selfishly, we create and contribute to dysfunctional relationships. Anytime we live selflessly, we create and contribute to functional relationships.

When we live selfishly, we are choosing sin. When we live selflessly, we are choosing godliness. Sin always impacts relationships negatively. Godliness always impacts relationships positively.

> Anytime we live selfishly, we create and contribute to dysfunctional relationships.

As you are pursuing a healthy you, it would be a great advantage in your spiritual and relational fitness to live selflessly. Healthy relationships occur only when we live selflessly. This is not easy, but it is something we must do.

How to Live Selflessly

There are three ways I want to share that each of us can live more selflessly.

1. Die daily to self.

We should strive to live out Galatians 2:19-20. It says, "For through the law I died to the law, so that I might live for God. I have been crucified with Christ, and I no longer live, but Christ lives in me. The life I now live in the body, I live by faith in the Son of God, who loved me and gave himself for me." At the Jerusalem council, the question was, "How is a person really saved?" Paul declares that we are either saved by the law and our works, or we are saved by God's grace.[2]

Salvation by the Law is impossible. We cannot work our way up to heaven. Salvation is in Christ alone. We are saved by Christ alone and His miraculous grace.

This is pivotal to accurately understanding and interpreting Galatians 2:19-20. Paul declared, "I have been crucified with Christ." The apostle Paul believed that he was crucified with Christ when he repented of his sin and placed his faith in Christ alone for his salvation. This is when Paul began dying to self daily. I agree one hundred percent, because this is the Word of God. The moment we repent of our sin and place our faith in Christ alone, we are crucified with Christ. We choose, at that moment, death to self and life with God.

From salvation on, I no longer live to fulfill my personal rights and desires. Why is this so? Because Christ lives in me, and He is the hope of glory. Colossians 1:27 states, "Christ in you, the hope of glory." This entry into a new relationship with God is marked by fellowship with Jesus Christ. This is now the life I live as long as I breathe. How do I do this? By faith alone in Christ alone! This is my new life and the new way I live daily. Jesus loved me and gave Himself for me for this cause. Therefore, fellowship with God occurs. This is only possible with a positive response to all Jesus did for me on the cross.

Moreover, this truth—that we are crucified with Christ—marks a life in which we die to ourselves daily. Daily we deny self, take up our cross, and follow Jesus.

I find it helpful as I start each day with God to declare what God says about me already: *I have been crucified with Christ.* This is a living truth that reminds me that dead people have no rights. I am now a dead man to my old self and my past way of living. Jesus changed it all. I have no rights. I belong only to Him. This new way is a selfless way.

Now that you have a greater understanding of this selfless way for each of us to live, standing on the authority of Scripture, you choose to live selflessly. Now you are ready.

Pray daily and tell God passionately: *Lord, I want to live selflessly.*

2. Walk away from control.

Since we realize we are crucified with Christ and have absolutely zero rights, we have to determine to do a very difficult thing: *Walk away from control.* Many of us who have the gift of leadership will struggle greatly with walking away from control.

The Christian life is not about me. The Christian life is living for Jesus in the way that He desires for me to live—selflessly.

Therefore, we need to walk away from the control of fighting needless battles. Every issue does not have to become a personal issue to defend or do. Every hill is not worth dying on. Walk away from needless battles.

We also need to walk away from thinking we should always have the last word in every conversation. Having the final word in every conversation can be destructive relationally. Be willing to walk away from always having the final word.

Additionally, we need to walk away from always thinking we are called to run the world and everyone's life in it. This is not easy for any of us, but in all reality, our hands are full with leading ourselves!

We are not called to run the entire world and everyone else's life. God is. Trust Him. Live selflessly.

3. Initiate relationships.

Be willing to take the first step in relationships. When a person is selfish, they think that people should come to them. We need to become not just responsive to others, but pro-active in our relationships and in the formulation of new relationships.

In a relationship that has become dysfunctional, be sure you initiate repentance and forgiveness, doing whatever needs to be done to make it right. The more you live selflessly, the more you will initiate and engage in relationships.

In order to live fit relationally, you have to live selflessly. This is not easy to do. Without dying to ourselves daily, walking away from control, and having productive, flourishing relationships in life, we will find it very difficult to live selflessly.

Choose God's way. Live selflessly.

CHAPTER 10
Live Lovingly

As followers of Christ, we are on a major pursuit to find out what God wants us to do with our life and discover how to get it done. God wants us to love Him and to love others. Love travels on the tracks of a relationship.

At times, we are like a team who knows we need to score more points but does not know how. Or maybe we are like a government that knows we need to deal with financial challenges in our nation, but just doesn't know the best approach. As we live out our faith in all areas of life, there are times and situations we are just like these examples. We know what God wants, but we are just not sure how to get it done.

The great news is that in this chapter, we will discover together that it is more than clear what God wants us to do: *Love Him and love other people.* Furthermore, we will learn some ways He wants us to do this practically and effectively.

Everything else in your life will be influenced by how you live out what will be shared here. You want to get this right. If you do not, sooner or later, there will be a price to pay that will negatively impact each of the other areas of your life.

Being fit relationally hinges on understanding what God wants and how He wants us to love Him and love others. The challenge before us is to live lovingly.

The Greatest Need Before Us

There is so much conversation about our greatest needs in the workplace, in the church, and in all segments of America and the world. Conversations like these are healthy, but their value will only be as good as what is referenced as the basis of truth.

As you know, I believe in the authority and infallibility of the Holy Scripture in the Bible. This is my basis of truth. If God says it, it is truth.

> Being fit relationally hinges on understanding what God wants and how He wants us to love Him and love others.

Knowing this to be true and right, I think it is more than clear that our greatest need is to see a revival of the first and second greatest commandments found in the Scripture.

One day, an expert in the Law came to Jesus, trying to test Him. His question to Jesus was interesting and Jesus' response to His question is the heartbeat of our discussion in this chapter. The Scripture says in Matthew 22:36-40, "'Teacher, which command in the law is the greatest?' He said to him, 'Love the Lord your God with all your heart, with all your soul, and with all your mind. This is the greatest and most important command. The second is like it: Love your neighbor as yourself. All the Law and the Prophets depend on these two commands.'" What Jesus values, we need to value. This is not up for debate. *He is Truth and He tells the truth.*

The greatest need in each of us, in our families, in our places of work, in our churches, in sports, entertainment, education, media, law, and politics, as well as the greatest need in America and every part of this world is to live out what Jesus said in these verses: *Love God and love others.*

This is God's plan and God's will for each of us. *There is nothing greater than love.*

Going Deeper in Our Understanding

These profound words of Jesus Christ recorded in Matthew 22 have their deep roots in Deuteronomy 6:4-5, which states, "Listen, Israel: The LORD our God, the LORD is one. Love the LORD your God with all your heart, with all your soul, and with all your strength." Founded on a theological declaration that there is no one like the Lord our God because the Lord is one, we need to hear the plea of Deuteronomy 6 with the full intent to obey: *Love God!*

The Israelites were taught to repeat these words to their children continually, remind themselves of them constantly, and keep public records that contained and proclaimed them unashamedly. We need to catch the fire they had in their hearts about how important this command was to their faith and their relationships.

How does God want to be loved?

Let's go deeper and discover how we can live this out passionately.

1. Wholeheartedly

God's call to love Him is a call to commitment. This commitment is based upon much more than emotion or feeling, but on your personal devotion to Him. As God is placed and praised as your sole priority in your life, He wants you to love Him with all you are and all you have, wholeheartedly. Without any reservation, without holding anything back, love God wholeheartedly.

2. Intellectual intentionality

As we are called to love God with all our heart, we know this also means to love Him with intellectual intentionality. In Moses' day, the people of God believed that your heart was your intellect, and the call to love God required you to love Him with full intellectual understanding. Intellectual laziness was not applauded, and biblical illiteracy kept you from living like God desired. Therefore, you were to be intentional about understanding God.

Loving God wholeheartedly with the highest manner of intellectual intentionality needs to be rediscovered in our generation of Christianity. Passionlessness and laziness plague the testimony of Christianity today.

3. Entire being

God wants us to love Him with our entire being. We need to love Him with every part of who we are until we have nothing left.

I have a small figurine of a soldier coming home from the battles of the Civil War. With his horse looking exhausted and barely able to stand, the soldier is leaning forward over the horse, personifying what is described as *Nothing Left* by artist F. J. Barnum.

This is a clear picture of how we need to love God with our entire being. We are to love God with all we are, with all we have, and in all we do in life. People should never be able to tell where Jesus ends and we begin because there is such oneness with Him.

4. Dynamic energy

As you love God wholeheartedly, with a commitment to intellectual intentionality so you can love Him with your entire being, you are to do so with dynamic energy. Loving God with all your strength means to love Him with a powerful, compelling, contagious, and dynamic energy. We are to love Him for who He is and with all we are.

Families, churches, workplaces, schools, politics, towns, cities, and all of America and the world will be impacted like never before in our generation when we begin to love God like He demands and deserves to be loved.

How God Loves You

God has shown how He loves us through the grace given to us through the sacrificial death of Jesus Christ for our sin. His amazing grace removes our sin completely.

The way God wants to be loved as I have described in the above section is still not representative of the way God loves each of us. How does God love us?

I want to highlight these compelling ways that I believe and know God loves you:

- **Willfully:** God so loved you He willfully gave His Son, Jesus Christ for you.[1] No one made God do it. He is God! He loves you because He wants to love you.
- **Sacrificially:** Jesus gave His life to die on the cross for your sins. He sacrificed Himself for you and me. He died in our place. He became the perfect, once and for all sacrifice for our sins.[2]
- **Unconditionally:** God loves you regardless of how you live, how you conduct yourself, and how you treat Him and others. He loves you unconditionally.[3] As much as and in the same way that He loves you, He loves the drunk on the street, the homeless man cuddled up in a blanket on a park bench, the drug addict close to an overdose, and the meanest person you know . . . unconditionally.

How to Love Other People

When God calls you to love your neighbor as you love yourself, it is a big call, and it's placed upon every person. There is one thing we definitely do well: love ourselves.

We sing *How Great We Are* much more than we sing *How Great Thou Art*.

So, how do we love people? How does God want us to love people? God wants us to love people the same way He loves us. How are you doing loving other people in these ways?

- **Willfully:** Our love for God should be so great that we want to love other people willfully. We should not have to be asked to show a person love and care during a bad time in their life. We should not have to work up to caring for other people. Our love for other people should happen willfully, naturally, and genuinely.

- **Sacrificially:** Love other people like Jesus loved you. Sacrificial love is giving up your own self for the sake of someone else. The call of Jesus to love others sacrificially is convicting. His words are more than sufficient to describe this to us. Read these next words slowly. Then read them again. Jesus said as recorded in John 15:12-13, "This is my command: Love one another as I have loved you. No one has greater love than this: to lay down his life for his friends."

- **Unconditionally:** Since Jesus loves us unconditionally, we need to love others in the same way. Regardless of how they treat us and how they live, it is our responsibility to love all people unconditionally. Even if their lifestyle is extremely far away from God's will and intention, love them unconditionally. While you hold the truth of God in one hand, you hold the love of God in the other. God's truth and loving people are never contradictory, but always complimentary. Love all people unconditionally. In all levels of relationships with other people, love them willfully, sacrificially, and unconditionally.

The Greatest Lesson I Ever Learned about Love

It was the late 1980s. God was blessing us immeasurably. Our church was buzzing and growing. God was moving powerfully. We had just moved into a new worship center and transition was taking place. While our numbers were gaining, we also saw a few individuals and families depart. As any pastor and leader would be, I was troubled.

God raised up a man to walk with me through these days of transition. His name was Ron Lewis, and he was so helpful to me. After listening to me talk about a few departures we had during that transition time, I will never forget what Ron told me.

Sitting in a back room of an old Bonanza restaurant, working through how we could sustain the momentum of our church, Ron looked at me and said, *"Ronnie, never let anyone outside of your circle of love."* When I heard those words, I felt God had given them directly to me through Ron.

Ron continued, developing and expounding on his remark to me. He shared that if my heart was big enough to forgive continually and love unconditionally, I could continue a relationship with individuals and families regardless of where they went to church, and even if they left the church I was called to pastor. Even today, I hear those words resounding continually, *"Ronnie, never let anyone outside of your circle of love."*

Even though I was a young leader, I took Ron's counsel to heart immediately. In the days following, God did a major work in my life personally and as a pastor.

Beginning on that day, I have done my best to never let anyone outside of my circle of love. I do not have the right to love one person but not another. Jesus sets the bar high: love all people! Yes, love all people unconditionally. Through life daily, within your family and outside of your family, including the workplace and the church, always practice this: *Never let anyone outside of your circle of love.*

How You Live This Out

Before we bring closure in this chapter, these are some ways I have found we can live out the commitment to never let anyone outside of our circle of love:

- **Take people to the Lord in prayer:** People will hurt you and even offend you deeply. Others will lie about you and cause problems for you. A few may even walk out of your life. Take each one of them to the Lord in prayer by name. There is no need to talk to other people about them. Talk to God about them.

- **Forgive continually:** Forgiveness is a way of life. Unforgiveness is not a friend to you, so do not cuddle up to it. Do not try to turn this rattlesnake of unforgiveness into your pet or friend. If you do, it will strike you with a poison that will eventually destroy you. Unforgiveness and bitterness never have a place in the life of a Christian. Love and forgiveness always win.

- **Let it go:** Regardless of what has been said about you, done to you, written about you, or presumed about you, let it go. Take it to the Lord in prayer. Forgive continually. Then, let it go! You cannot go forward holding on to a past hurt. You cannot go forward resenting people or situations. I know how difficult this can be, but you must realize that holding on to the past is spiritually and relationally unhealthy. Let it go!

Choosing to never let anyone outside of my circle of love has been the greatest personal lesson I have ever learned about love. What is yours?

Knowing all that is in this chapter, it is truly a challenge for each of us daily. Love God. Love others. Live your life lovingly.

CHAPTER 11

Live Connecting

Love travels on the tracks of relationship.[1] Your life will never become any greater than the relationships you have. It is impossible to love others like God loves without having a relationship with them. Love *does* travel on the tracks of relationship.

Living fit relationally is absolutely critical to making your life count by pursuing a healthy you. While connecting with people will help you personally, there is nothing that will improve your life like connecting with a spiritual community. I am convinced that relational fitness occurs much more effectively when you are connected to a spiritual community, a local church.

You May Go Faster, But Never Farther

We live in a culture that is ignited by traveling at a rapid pace. While coupling pace with the passion of "doing your own thing" may be exciting, it often leads to danger.

At times, you may go faster in life when you go alone, but you will never go farther. This is why you need to be connected to a local church.

Planting your life in and living your life with a vibrant, enthusias-
tic, spiritual community will do more for you than you can imagine.
If you have the privilege of being part of this kind of spiritual family
today, you already know this.

A local church cannot live your life for you, but the church can
live life with you. The church is not a building; it is the people—the
community of believers. Connecting to a local spiritual community
will ignite you to live more effectively and consistently.

This is why I am convinced that you may go faster at times in
your life when you go alone, but you will never go farther.

What Jesus Values, We Should Also Value

Jesus places high value on His Church. The Scripture is clear
that Jesus died for His Church. There is not a higher price to pay
than to give one's life. Clearly, Jesus loves the Church.

When the apostle Paul was giving instructions about marriage
to the church of Ephesus, he also gave us an incredible insight
into the church and how Jesus feels about it. Ephesians 5:23 says,
"Christ is the head of the church. He is the Savior of the body." Then
he goes on with a challenge to the people. In Ephesians 5:25, in a
word to the spiritual leader of the family, the husband, he states,
"Husbands, love your wives, just as Christ loved the church and
gave himself for her."

Without any question, Jesus places high value on His Church.
Jesus says He is the head of the Church, not some man on this
earth. Jesus is the Savior of the body, no one else. Jesus is the
only Savior of the world. Then Paul states something I find absolutely amazing. He declares that Jesus loved the Church and gave
Himself for her. Why? Jesus loves the Church willfully, sacrificially,
and unconditionally. He values the Church and so should we.

But that is not all. Even Jesus Himself stated, as recorded in Matthew 16:18, "And I also say to you that you are Peter, and on this rock I will build my church, and the gates of Hades will not overpower it." Jesus claims that He owns the Church. The church is Jesus' Church. It is not anyone else's church. Jesus is the only one who died for the Church and paid the price for us.

Jesus gives the highest value to the Church. He owns the Church. He is the Head of the Church. He died for the Church. He is one day coming back to this earth again for His Church. Jesus values the Church in the highest way.

We should do the same.

Why Connecting with a Church Is Important

If you are going to live connecting, you should not only live connecting with God daily, but also connecting with a local church at least weekly. Let's look at why connecting with a local church is so important.

1. Connecting with a local church is the biblical thing to do.

When the Bible speaks, God speaks. Therefore, whatever God says, He means. The Bible is not a fantasy or a fairy tale. The Bible is the absolute authority for life, faith, and practice. It is by the Bible that we should live our lives.

When you read the New Testament, you are reading a historical record of God's activity in the Church. You are also reading letters that have been written to specific local churches. These churches are even referred to by their names.

For example, here are some of the churches who are specifically called by name in the New Testament:

- Philippians 1:1: "To all the saints in Christ Jesus who are in Phillipi."

- Romans 1:7: "To all who are in Rome, loved by God, called as saints."
- Ephesians 1:1: "To the faithful saints in Christ Jesus at Ephesus."

Beyond these, many others are mentioned in the New Testament.

What does this illustrate? It shows us that while the entire book of Acts is a historical record of the Church in its earliest days, the epistles in the New Testament were written to specific churches, often mentioning people in the churches by name. These letters to New Testament churches reveal that living as a part of a church is the norm for Christians. The New Testament authors always assume that Christians will be connected to a local church.

2. Connecting with a local church is a personal thing to do.

Those Christians who disregard the Church need to go back to the Bible and read it again. For example, did you know that the word *members* is used connected to the Church? First Corinthians 12:27 states, "Now you are the body of Christ, and individual members of it." The word *members* in this passage is a reference to body parts, saying that each Christian is to be a part of the body of the local church.

In fact, when you look at the entire chapter of 1 Corinthians 12, you see how each member is important and has been assigned a specific role within the body of Christ. Their specific role is related to the spiritual gifts that have been given to them at salvation by the Holy Spirit.

In order to rightly illustrate individual members being mentioned, notice that in Philippians it mentions Clement, Euodia, and Syntyche. In 1 Corinthians, Phoebe is mentioned as a dynamic believer in the church at Cenchrea. In Acts, Priscilla and Aquila were mentioned by name, as well as in 1 Corinthians, Romans, and

1 Timothy. They are referenced as great leaders in the church. This list goes on and on.

Ministry in and through a local church travels on the tracks of relationship. We see this modeled all through the churches in the New Testament. The Church of today needs to recapture this idea, because this is God's ideal.

3. Connecting with a local church is the wise thing to do.

If you want to be fit relationally, I can assure you the wisest thing you can do is connect with a local church. The skeptics and cynics would say that the Church is full of hypocrites. I am sure that may have a grain of truth in it; after all, the Church is full of sinners. But it's full of forgiven sinners, being made more like Jesus.

While local churches are not perfect, they are biblical and full of members who connect at least once a week for worship and to live life together. If you want to go further in your life, connect with a church. It is the wisest thing you can do.

Why is it wise to become part of a local spiritual family, a local church? I hope you will consider these reasons.

Through the local church, you can be equipped to live your life on mission with God. The pastor of a local church has been charged to equip the saints to do the work of the ministry. God wants to use each person in the Church to live life on mission with God. Whether you are in corporate America, politics, entertainment, sports, education, media, a stay-at-home parent, or vocational ministry, you need to live life on mission with God. This gives you an opportunity to be part of something that is bigger than yourself.

Through the local church, unity in the midst of diversity can be portrayed to the entire world. Sadly, the culture is full of racial injustice, cultural debates, and great division. The local church should be the most diverse representation of the entire community in which you serve. Not just diversity relating to ethnicity, but to various cultural backgrounds, where people are from, and how they live presently. Additionally, there can be a diversity of leaders, who will not all think and look alike, but share the common mission of making disciples to reach the world for Jesus Christ. For you personally, being engaged in a local church can increase your appreciation for all persons regardless of the color of their skin, the difficulties of their past, and their present or current challenges. This is another reason that your connection to a local church is the wisest thing to do.

Through the local church, ministry may also occur in your community, across America, and even throughout the world. Local churches have the ability to shape their communities because of their capacity to meet the needs of people by caring for the needy, visiting the sick, meeting the needs of widows, ministering to those in prison, and even helping some of these people re-enter society effectively. This is a small list of ministries in which most healthy churches have some direct involvement. Being part of a church that is highly committed to ministry in their community can help ascend your future spiritually and relationally.

When you are connected to a local church and your pastor is preaching and teaching the Bible as the Word of God for your life, this will help you make wise decisions personally. Decision-making in all areas of life can be complex and challenging. But when you are under the teaching of God's Word weekly, God will use His Word to impart wisdom that is needed for each decision with which you are faced. As a bonus, if you are still in need of assistance, you can connect with your pastor and he can guide you in seeking God's wisdom.

It is through a local church that your family can find added value for your lives. Each member of your family, regardless of their age, can find value in and through the local church. You need things in your life that add value to you personally and to your family. The church can! The church does! It also adds value to the community and to the world. The church does this in ways no one else can.

Through the local church, you can rest with confidence knowing you do not have to walk through life alone. The church is there for you and with you. Every person will walk through major challenges in life. They will lose people around them to death. They will grieve. They will get sick. They will have surgery. A few may lose their jobs and face a crisis in identity like they never have before. Regrettably, some marriages will end in divorce.

When you are an active part of a church, you do not have to walk through these times alone. In fact, you will probably meet and be ministered to by others who have suffered a similar challenge or loss. Choose not to walk alone in life. Live life with the church.

> Through the local church, you can rest with confidence knowing you do not have to walk through life alone.

I believe that each person who knows Jesus Christ as Savior and Lord needs to live tightly connected to the Church. You need to be connected because it is the biblical thing to do, a personal thing to do and the wise thing to do.

Live Connecting

I hope you will live your life connecting with God daily. I pray you will live your life connecting with other people daily. I am convinced there is a huge need to live connecting to a local church.

I am not talking about dropping into a worship service once every eight weeks. I am talking about buying in by giving one year of your life to see all God will do if you are highly engaged with a local church at least once weekly. I am convinced it will change your life and perspective completely. You may not notice the difference immediately. In fact, it may seem inconvenient at first. But twenty years later, I believe you will be able to look back and think, *when I took the challenge to do all my church asked me to do for one year, it changed my life and trajectory, not only for my own future, but for my family.* Being fit relationally becomes a reachable goal when you are engaged in a dynamic local church at least once a week. There is something special about being connected with a local church. There is nothing like it.

As I stated earlier in this chapter, *you may go faster at times in your life when you go alone, but you will never go further.* This is why you need to be connected to a local church. Live connecting.

CHAPTER 12
Live Serving

In the game of tennis, the serve is the most important shot. It positions you for the rest of the game. When your serve is on, you have a mental edge in the game. The better your serve, the bigger the weapon you have against your opponent. Your chances of winning the match increase greatly if your serve is highly effective.

Serving always begins the game of tennis, but life is a little different. Sometimes we are able to project a need before it exists and initiate service. Other times, we respond in order to meet a need once it already exists.

Teams, companies, groups, and churches are at their very best when they are serving. Just as it is in tennis, you increase your chances to win when you are serving effectively.

What I Have Observed through the Years

Northwest Arkansas has been my home for the last thirty years. It is also the global headquarters of Walmart, J. B. Hunt, Tyson Foods, and the University of Arkansas. Beyond being filled with outstanding private businesses, large and small, with thriving leaders and an explosive real estate market, it also has more than fourteen hundred national and international companies that have a presence here to serve their Walmart account. These companies, known as vendors of Walmart, employ anywhere from a few people to several hundred.

The University of Arkansas adds to this energetic and thriving region. The presence of a major, growing university gives sparks of life and vitality to a region that is already robust with a strong business community. Needless to say, for those of us who have lived in this region for a while, this is not the Northwest Arkansas that existed ten years ago. Things have changed dramatically.

What I have observed over the years is the growing presence of leaders. They abound in this region more than ever before. This entire region was initially built through dynamic leadership, and it is continuing to attract leaders.

What I have also observed in this region are the outstanding people who have served these organizations, businesses, and cities so humbly and effectively. While only a few people get their names mentioned in the media, this robust climate is energized by countless willing people who want to serve and make a difference with their lives. Some serve on farms, in warehouses, or drive trucks; others are in office complexes marketing their products or serving their customer's needs. These companies are winning because their people are serving effectively.

What I have also observed in this region is the transition to a new kind of person and leader. I have witnessed, up close, an entire global company turn around in their trajectory through servant leadership. From the top to the bottom of the organization, servant leadership was championed. Servant leadership was not just an aspiration or empty talk; it became a reality visible to all.

Serving others always results in a healthy relationship. Therefore, live serving.

What Ignites Service

Discovering and developing who you are spiritually, physically, and relationally will ignite you to a life of service. When you are spiritually fit, physically fit, and relationally fit, serving others becomes a natural and healthy part of your life.

> **Serving others always results in a healthy relationship.**

Jesus Christ modeled a life of service. Everywhere He went and through everything He did, Christ personified serving.

Humility was a way of life for Jesus. From being born in a stable to identifying with everyone in His life, and never playing favorites, humility is chiseled into the life of Jesus. Society scorned the Son of God. He was executed on a cross, dying in total and complete humility. Jesus personified humility and service.

Within the final few days of Jesus' life, He did something with His disciples and friends that still captivates us today. Jesus loved His disciples and friends to the end. With the cross looming before Him, His focus was still on these who were with Him.

We read this story in John 13:4-5: "So he got up from supper, laid aside his outer clothing, took a towel, and tied it around himself. Next, he poured water into a basin and began to wash his disciples' feet and to dry them with the towel tied around him."

While the cultural practice was that a servant would wash the feet of a dinner guest before eating, on this evening Jesus washed the feet of those who had walked with Him throughout the last three years of His life.

Initially, Peter absolutely refused to let Jesus wash His feet. At that point, Jesus told Peter he would have no part with Him. Peter was stunned. Then Peter—in his typical fashion—told Jesus that if this was so, Jesus should wash not only his feet, but also his hands and his head! Peter wanted all of Jesus, not just part of Him.

Jesus served the Father that night by washing all of His disciples' feet, including Judas Iscariot. Jesus loved him unconditionally and served him sacrificially, even knowing all the time Judas was to soon betray Him.

Because Jesus had such an intimate relationship with His Father, He served others with humility. It was not forced. It was who He was from the inside out.

When we are fit, we will serve others with humility. When we choose humility and service, we choose to be like Jesus. When we are willing to meet even the most basic needs, we are serving with humility.

Could this be our greatest service to God?

Pride promotes self, service promotes others. Pride is a selfish choice, service is an unselfish choice. Pride is dangerous, service is life-giving. Pride brings people down, service lifts people up.

You will never make your life count when life is all about you. This is unhealthy. Relational health occurs when you are serving others. All of this is ignited because you are relationally fit.

How to Develop Your Serve

Tennis players work on their serve constantly. The more effective their serve, the greater the probability for them to win. They have not only been coached in their serving, they also continually work to develop it.

As Christ followers, we must continually practice serving God and others. Being a servant and serving the Lord and others is important to us because it was important in the life of Jesus and the New Testament Church.

In Thom S. Rainer's book, *I Am a Church Member*, he states: "The word *servant* occurs fifty-seven times in the New Testament. Sometimes it refers to a person who has that official role in a household. But many times it refers to the role we are to assume as Christians. Also, *serve* occurs fifty-eight times in the New Testament. Get the picture? Serving is important in the Bible."[1]

As followers of Jesus Christ, we need to be much more committed to improving our service to the Lord and others than any tennis player would be in developing their serve.

We can learn from Jesus. His life was marked by humility and service. None of us are servants naturally. We can only become servants of God and to others supernaturally.

> As Christ followers, we must continually practice serving God and others.

What can we do to develop our serve? How can we see the serving spirit resonate in and through our own lives? Consider these four major ways to develop your serve.

1. Become spiritually fit.

The more spiritually fit you are, the greater the probability that serving will emerge in your life. You cannot separate the intensity and intentionality of your personal walk with Christ from your own personal commitment to serving others.

The more Jesus is doing in you, the more Jesus will do through you. His work within you will change you from the inside out. None of us can work up love or work up to service. Both have to flow from who you are in Christ. Yes, from the inside out.

Therefore, I am convinced the greatest way each of us can develop a serving spirit and humble attitude is to walk closely with Jesus Christ. The more we are with Jesus, the more we will look like Jesus. His legacy of service has been and will be unmatched forever.

2. Become motivated by others who serve.

Studying people who excel in an area of their life always motivates me. For example, think about a few people the apostle Paul commended for their service.

In Colossians 4:7 we read, "Tychicus, our dearly loved brother, faithful minister, and fellow servant in the Lord, will tell you all the news about me." While Paul had some enemies, he also had friends like Tychicus. Paul loved him like a brother and he was his spiritual brother in Christ. He regarded him as a "fellow servant," a term at times translated "fellow bond-servant in the Lord." He served Christ with Paul and often delivered news and even letters for Paul like Colossians, Ephesians, and Philemon. As a loyal friend to Paul, Tychicus must also have been a man who walked with God intimately and passionately.

In Colossians 4:12, Paul states these words about a man named Epaphras: "Epaphras, who is one of you, a servant in Christ Jesus, sends you greetings. He is always wrestling for you in his prayers, so that you can stand mature and fully assured in everything God wills." This is a dynamic testimony about a man who was saved in Ephesus and was used by God to start the church in Colossae. He was a mighty prayer warrior, and was called by his friend Paul "a servant in Christ Jesus."

Men like Epaphras and Paul saw themselves as slaves of Christ. It was a badge of honor for them. They were even prisoners at one time together, all for the sake of Christ. Above all, Epaphras served Jesus, but he also served the Church by praying like few other intercessors and served with his friend Paul.

If these two do not motivate you enough, think about Luke. In Colossians 4:14, Paul calls Luke "the dearly loved physician." Luke served Paul not only as his physician, but also as the writer who recorded the entire book of Acts and his own account of the gospel of Jesus Christ. Luke was with Paul so much in his travels, he referred to them as "we" in the book of Acts. Luke was truly unique in his service. He used his giftedness to serve the Lord, to serve Paul, and to serve the Church.

Men like Tychicus, Epaphras, Luke, and Paul motivate me to serve others and to serve the Lord. Each served because of a deep passion for Christ.

3. Become connected to a local church.

Being in a vibrant, growing, Bible-based church that is committed to reaching its own community can do so much to develop our service to God and others. There are so many ways to serve in the Church.

The Church needs to become the greatest development center for servant leaders in the world today. We cannot just develop leaders; we must develop servant leaders. Any genuine servant is always influencing others and organizations through their serving spirit, even if they don't receive any praise for doing so.

Something happens in us and begins to happen through us when we are connected to a church that serves the Lord and others. As God begins to stir your heart to serve, to give of yourself for the sake of others and the gospel of Christ, there is no telling how you will find yourself serving through your church, in your community, in our nation, or even across the world.

4. Become engaged in serving.

Go ahead and dive in! Becoming engaged in serving sparks further service to the Lord and others. Nothing turns on your spiritual jets more than serving others.

As a pastor, I could probably rationalize my life and say all I do is serve the Lord and others. Maybe it seems that way from a big-picture view, even though it still sounds like a stretch. But here is what I know. When I am engaged in officiating a funeral, ministering to a grieving family, praying for someone in the hospital, performing a marriage ceremony for a couple I love, winning someone to Jesus Christ, or somewhere in the midst of deep, missional engagement, I am greatly energized.

Becoming engaged in serving leads to more serving. Leading others is serving, but serving those you lead faithfully takes your influence to an entirely new level.

The greatest and most influential leaders I have known have been servant leaders. When evaluating the entire person, each is

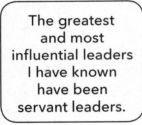

The greatest and most influential leaders I have known have been servant leaders.

a genuine servant leader who lives and leaves legacies that are indelible. People can change the world through servant leadership.

Serving God is the greatest thing you can do in your life. This is not limited by vocation, only by your heart.

Serving others is what God wants you to do with your life. Serving is not limited to what you do through a community initiative or a mission trip somewhere in the world. Serving needs to become who you are and be carried out wherever you are. Do not limit what God may want to do through you.

Being fit spiritually and even being fit physically will have a major impact on being fit relationally. When you are physically fit and as healthy as you can be, you will have more energy to serve the Lord and others.

The greater you serve, the more you will be positioned to make the biggest impact with your life. Change your world through serving God and serving others. Live serving.

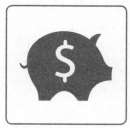

SECTION 4

Living Fit Financially

CHAPTER 13

Live Wisely

 Wisdom is seeing life from God's perspective. I need God's perspective about every area in my life. We all do.

The only way we receive God's wisdom is to live by what God says in the Bible. We need the light of God's Word to illuminate our way. Psalm 119:105 says, "Your word is a lamp for my feet and a light on my path." This verse clearly states why we need God's perspective and wisdom.

There is a major problem in America today that crosses all generations and ethnicities. God's wisdom and perspective on this problem are needed now more than ever before. *This major problem is how people handle money.*

How you choose to handle money will either ascend or sink your life. How financially fit are you?

Many people can check the boxes in a positive way:

- Spiritually fit: Check!
- Physically fit: Check!
- Relationally fit: Check!

But when they come to being financially fit, they *cannot* check.

LIVING FIT

Usually, financial challenges are not isolated. They affect and are affected by all areas of life. You may want to work through those boxes again after you read this chapter.

Financial troubles create enormous pressure in life. Even more so, these financial troubles create major relational challenges among families and employees.

Financial challenges drain you emotionally and completely distort your vision. I have seen it bring a person down not just spiritually, but also physically. I have seen a person who was once so positive and optimistic about life and business, turn into being negative and pessimistic about everything. I have seen couples, once so happy together, become deeply resentful toward each other.

Through the years, I have witnessed extremely wealthy people go through financial challenges and, in some cases, lose it all. I have also observed average income people and families living paycheck-to-paycheck, juggling bill after bill, seeing no hope for their financial future. This reminds each of us that it is not about how much money you have or how much money you do not have. It comes down to one thing: *How you handle money.* Your perspective determines how you handle money. This is why we need God's perspective in life.

This section of the book will call each of us to living fit financially. The challenges we are addressing are real challenges and each one of us needs help relating to them.

Will you join us in this journey? Don't just read about financial fitness; act upon it. Determine now, once and for all, from this day forward that you will . . .

- Live Wisely
- Live Responsibly
- Live Generously
- Live Indelibly

I believe if you will take this section seriously, the direction of your life, family, and future will change forever.

It's Bad

We have all been in those situations when we knew the news was not going to be good. Going in, we ask, "How bad is it?" Someone looks at us and says, "It's bad."

We are entering into the subject about finances with the same trepidation. How bad is it? It's bad.

We know this, so I will give just a few sentences here to help us understand its severity. Consider these facts:

- Fifty-nine percent of divorcees say finances played a major role in the breakup of their marriage.[1]
- $179,806 is the average mortgage debt.[2]
- $49,042 is the average student loan debt by household.[3]
- $16,061 is the average credit card debt.[4]
- U.S. citizens spend $1.26 for every $1 they earn.[5]
- There is $1.3 trillion of student loan debt in America.[6]
- There is $1 trillion of credit card debt in America.[7]
- $20 trillion is the national debt of the United States.[8]
- Eighty percent of the small businesses that open fail in the first five years. The primary reason they fail is financial problems.[9]

This list of statistics could easily get longer, but I think you get the picture. Yes, it's bad.

These challenges drain you emotionally and completely distort your vision. When this happens to a single person, it's threatening, but for families, it can be devastating.

We need wisdom. How do we move into a healthier position financially? How do we live wisely?

5 Principles for Winning with Money Over Time

In March of 2017, I began a weekly podcast about life and leadership. Each week, I interview one of the great leaders in America about helping people live well and coaching people to become great leaders. For twenty-two minutes a week, anyone who wants to be encouraged about life and leadership can listen to our podcast.

One of my first podcasts was with Dave Ramsey of Ramsey Solutions. For more than twenty-five years, Dave has been teaching people how to handle money. He does so through his radio broadcasts all over the nation, with millions of weekly listeners. Ramsey Solutions provides biblically based, common sense education and empowerment that give HOPE to everyone in every walk of life.[10]

In my interview with Dave, I asked him for some principles that would help people handle money more wisely. I want to share these principles, or things to do, with you. They are relevant for everyone, from those who are trying to make it from paycheck to paycheck, to the wealthiest in the world. From the Bible, Dave has found these five principles:

1. *Be on a budget:* Develop a budget on paper and on purpose before each month begins.
2. *Get out of debt:* The borrower is slave to the lender all the time.
3. *Save money:* Wise people save money.
4. *High quality relationships:* You become who you hang around, and that affects your money.
5. *Generosity:* Outrageous generosity is correlated with winning with money.[11]

How does one improve upon these and other strategies Dave Ramsey has discovered through the years?

As you are pursuing a healthy you, you cannot be healthy if your finances are questionable. I think your financial fitness is just like your fitness physically and relationally. If any of these are not all they can be, it is a reflection upon your spiritual fitness. However, your past choices are past. Now you can begin to make future choices that can influence your entire life positively. Your present circumstances may now be beyond your control due to a few of these past choices, but God can give you a resolve to be faithful as you progress to your future. As your spiritual life goes, so goes the rest of your life.

This does not mean you cannot change your current financial path. Conversely, it means that you need to consider that everything in your life flows from your spiritual walk with Jesus Christ. Start there and line your life up by what the Bible says. This is what it means to be fit!

Fit does not mean you are perfect. Fit means you are working in your life, continually becoming all God wants you to become spiritually, physically, relationally, financially, and emotionally. Start where you are right now and work toward becoming healthy in each of these areas.

> Fit does not mean you are perfect. Fit means you are working in your life, continually becoming all God wants you to become.

You cannot control your past, but you can get on a new path toward your future. Your goal should be to become as healthy as you can be from this point on in each of these five areas of life.

Whatever your personal situation is financially, it does not alter what God's Word says. Your life should adjust to what God says, even about money. If a person or a family can avoid the traps of poor financial decision-making and management, they can pretty well beat the odds on other issues that come their way.

Insights about Money

As you keep in mind these five principles about money from bestselling author Dave Ramsey, I want to give you a few personal insights about money. When I was working on my doctorate degree, I did my main dissertation about money and finances. This has served as a biblical and theological basis that I have operated from personally. From this foundation, I have deep convictions about money because of what I learned decades ago and have tried to practice through the years.

- Money never satisfies.
- Money leads to worry.
- Money kept is money lost.
- Money cannot be taken to heaven or to hell.
- Money pursued for money's sake is like chasing after the wind.
- Money is a gift from God.

These truths can be found in Ecclesiastes 5:10–20, and paired with the insights already shared.

As you read through this passage, consider that the word *vanity* is used thirty-seven times in the book of Ecclesiastes. It speaks about the difficulty of understanding life. Financially wealthy King Solomon, who wrote these words, was declaring that life, money, and fame in and of themselves, only produce emptiness.

My desire is to give you all the weaponry necessary to win with money in your life. Your view of money and the way you handle it are determined by one person: you. For the sake of clarity, all of this should depend on one thing: *What God says in the Bible about money.*

Your attitude about money determines so much about the way you view and handle it. Money is not the end, but a necessary means to an end to live your life. It is a tool that God has entrusted to you. It does not and should not rule you, but you should manage it wisely. What does this mean?

The Most Important Thing You Need to Know about Money

From my personal study in the Bible, I discovered what I believe is the most important thing you need to know about money. When you know this one thing, it absolutely transforms your perspective about God, yourself, and the money and resources He has entrusted to you. What is it?

I believe the most important thing you need to know about money is this: *God owns everything and you own absolutely nothing.* Did you get this? *God owns everything and you own absolutely nothing.*

This is foundational for all you believe and will practice regarding money and resources—not just dollars and cents, but your entire salary, bonuses, stock, property, investments, and inheritance.

> God owns everything and you own absolutely nothing.

Two Decisions That Will Impact Your Future and Finances

One bad choice usually leads to other bad choices. Poor decision-making related to money can cripple you. On the other hand, one good choice usually leads to other good decisions. Good decision-making can impact your future and finances in a very positive way.

Decision 1: Avoid debt.

Do everything you can to avoid debt. I love what Dave Ramsey says about debt: "You can wander into debt, but you cannot wander out of it."[12]

The Bible says in Proverbs 22:7, "The rich rule over the poor, and the borrower is a slave to the lender." This is inescapable. Borrowing money always makes one a slave to the lender.

Dave teaches several steps you can take to get out of debt. I would encourage you to listen to our podcast with Dave and then go to his website to learn more about steps you can take to eliminate debt, and perhaps one day, be free from all debt.[13]

If you are in debt, avoid future debt and work toward eliminating as much debt as possible. This is very important to living wisely.

Decision 2: Give God at least the first tenth of all He has entrusted to you.

The greatest decision you can make for your future and finances is to give God at least the first tenth of all He has entrusted to you through your local church on the first day of each week, Sunday. Start here. Regardless of the challenges you may face in finances, start here. This has to become a non-negotiable in your life. This is the floor of giving, not the ceiling.

Remember, it all belongs to God. He did not give you all you have to waste or throw away, but to use for His glory to advance His kingdom throughout the world. This is how to live wisely.

In this chapter, I have intentionally placed several principles, insights, and convictions into your hands that are necessary to practice if you are truly going to live wisely. Live life by God's Word, and do so by living it out God's way every day. When you do, you are on the path to live wisely.

CHAPTER 14

Live Responsibly

Regardless of where we find ourselves financially, we need to live responsibly. Whatever our level of assets, we need to manage and use them responsibly.

Being irresponsible financially will place your family on a rapid descent from any level of success you may be experiencing today. While your intention will never be to lose money, assets, and resources, irresponsibility in decision making will jeopardize any stability you may be enjoying today.

Financial problems create enormous pressure in life. Not only will they impair your vision, they will affect you relationally and emotionally. Nothing will choke the joy out of your life more than financial pressures and worries.

This chapter is a call to live responsibly. This means that you are answerable. This means that you understand you will give an account to someone else for your life and the decisions you make. On the contrary, irresponsibility means that you believe you are not answerable for your actions. Living responsibly is healthy, while living irresponsibly is unhealthy.

On this pursuit of a healthy you, a compelling call is coming forth. Pertaining to money, assets, and resources, wisdom is calling you to a renewed commitment to live responsibly. When money, assets, and resources are involved, the stakes are high. Therefore, live responsibly.

The Driving Force of Living Responsibly

For those of us who believe in the Bible and what it says, we realize the cherished place of theology. Theology is the study of God. Breaking down the word *theology* leads us to understand that not only is theology the study of God, but it is also words about God. From these words about God and the study of God, we get our view of life and the entire world.

Theology touches every part of life. This includes money, assets, and resources. What God says about these things within the bigger context of all He says in His Word shapes our lives greatly.

Our theology of stewardship should be driven by one major theological doctrine. I believe this is the doctrine of God, what scholars call "Theology Proper." Think about where the Bible began. Genesis 1:1 says, "In the beginning God created the heavens and the earth." God is the Creator of all people and things. Therefore, He owns everything. Another declaration that affirms this is made in Psalm 24:1. It says, "The earth and everything in it, the world and all its inhabitants, belong to the LORD." When God created all things and did so out of nothing, He did what no one else can do and what no one else will ever be able to do. Why? He is God. God owns everything.

This doctrine of God is also expounded in Psalm 50:12, which says, "If I were hungry, I would not tell you, for the world and everything in it is mine." God declares boldly, "The world and everything in it is mine." Yes, God owns everything. Haggai 2:8 says, "'The silver and gold belong to me'—this is the declaration of the LORD of Armies." God owns everything. At the risk of being redundant, let me state again: *God is the Creator and Owner of all things.*

But this gets even greater and more personal. Genesis 1:26 says, "Then God said, 'Let us make man in our image, according to our likeness. They will rule the fish of the sea, the birds of the sky, the livestock, the whole earth.'" After God created man He gave him the authority to rule over all creation.

The word *rule* is very important in this text. It comes from the Hebrew word *radah*, which means "I rule." It is used twenty-two times in the Old Testament and is always limited to human dominion. In other words, God has entrusted to man the task of ruling over all of His creation.

This is furthered in the New Testament. Luke 16:2 says, "So he called the manager in and asked, 'What is this I hear about you? Give an account of your management, because you can no longer be my manager.'" The word *management* is the Greek word *oikonomos*, which means "to be a manager of an estate or an inspector of goods."[1] *Management* is also translated "stewardship." Therefore, while God owns everything, we are called to manage it for Him responsibly.

Living responsibly is living in accountability to God for your life and how you are managing all that He entrusts to you. Each of us is responsible and accountable to God in our management or stewardship.

The driving force of living responsibly is the doctrine of God. God does not have to consult with anyone about anything. He is God. He is over all, in all, and through all. He is sovereign in and over everything.

Never forget that God owns everything, because He created everything. We have been given the task of watching

> The driving force of living responsibly is the doctrine of God.

over His creation. We are accountable to God for our management, or if you prefer, our stewardship in life.

Three Important Convictions for Living Responsibly

Driven by a deep and rich doctrine of God, I want to give you three important convictions you should have in order to live responsibly. Relating to money, assets, and resources, these three things, when acted upon by anyone, will either ascend your life or sink it in a speedy descent. These things flow from the deep convictions already shared in this chapter.

1. God is the owner of everything.

God has no needs. He owns everything. God is sovereign over everything. Personally, my doctrine of God is that He is all, owns all, knows all, and demands all. The more I believe this, the more it will impact my life daily and my decision-making about everything.

2. You are a manager and temporary keeper of everything.

As King David declared in 1 Chronicles 29:16, "LORD our God, all this wealth that we've provided for building you a house for your holy name comes from your hand; everything belongs to you." Even the wealthy King David knew and practiced a deep belief that God owned everything, and anything he gave to God's house and people was really a gift back to God.

If God has entrusted you with money, assets, and resources, then He has given you the power, by His Spirit, to steward it wisely. Every talent and gift, as well as all treasures, are given to us to manage temporarily. Faithfulness to God and His Word is living responsibly.

This leads to a profound insight and a stirring challenge in life: *God owns everything and you own absolutely nothing.* While I stated this truth previously, by now you should know why I believe it so passionately. I am convinced this is foundational to the way you manage and expend all the money, assets, and resources God has entrusted to you. We must be both faithful and responsible in every way. This is what a manager and steward does.

3. You are accountable to God.

Each of us is accountable to God daily. In the Garden of Eden, Adam and Eve failed in their stewardship. God told them specific things He wanted from them, but they chose to disobey. Immediately, they became accountable for their stewardship.

Living responsibly in our management and stewardship occurs in a greater way when we know that we are accountable to God. The moment we believe it is ours will be the moment we enter into the sin that happened in Eden—disobedience to God.

No one can hide or run away from Romans 14:12. It says, "So then, each of us will give an account of himself to God." These words are inescapable. We cannot run and try to hide like Adam and Eve did in the Garden of Eden. God found them. God will find us.

He will hold us accountable for everything, including the way we manage all the money, assets, and resources He has entrusted to us.

Knowing this should impact our decision-making greatly. Our deep respect for God demands our best.

Seven Suggestions That Will Help You Live Responsibly in Your Everyday Choices

Knowing the right things to believe and do is one thing, but choosing to live them out daily takes it to a whole new level. Our everyday choices show how committed we are to living like God wants us to live. Whether these choices seem small or big, insignificant or significant, each is important to God and represents what we believe about who He is. God wants us to manage properly everything He has entrusted to us.

Therefore, in closing this chapter, I want to do what I can to help you live responsibly through your everyday choices relating to money, assets, and resources. Here is a list of seven suggestions that will help you live responsibly through your everyday choices.

1. Learn everything you can about what God says about money.

Ignorance in today's world about money, assets, and resources is unacceptable. Educate yourself in God's Word and God's ways about money. Money is not the end, but a means to an end. Money is a tool God has entrusted to you. Learn everything you can about the purpose of money: giving money, saving money, and spending money.

2. Develop a financial plan.

Whether your total resources are minimal or plentiful, develop a financial plan for your future. When you plan for failure, the outcome will soon follow. When you refuse to think about practical matters like monthly expenses, healthcare, life insurance, and retirement, you are living irresponsibly. You cannot declare that God will take care of you when you live without financial diligence.

3. Continually adjust your attitude.

Continually adjusting your attitude is very important. Otherwise you will slip into thinking "It's my money!", and you will arrogantly live this belief out. This is an unbiblical and improper view of money. It is not your money. It is God's money. Therefore, do not fall into this practice. Believing it is your money will lead to pain. You will reap what you sow. Continually adjust your attitude. Refuse to fall into the use of this verbiage and false belief about yourself. Remember, God owns everything and you own absolutely nothing.

4. Live on cash, not credit cards.

A credit mentality is a destructive mentality. If you play now, thinking credit is yours, you will pay later horribly and miserably. You are not financially healthy if you are living on credit. Sooner or later you will have to pay for it. The cost can be high and very painful.

> When you plan for failure, the outcome will soon follow. When you refuse to think about practical matters like monthly expenses, healthcare, life insurance, and retirement, you are living irresponsibly.

Credit card debt is the worst kind of debt. If you use a credit card, pay it off at the end of the month, every month. Many financial leaders and teachers like Dave Ramsey would say to cut up your credit cards and throw them in the trash.

5. Eliminate debt.

Strong warnings exist in Scripture relating to debt. Proverbs 6 tells us if we are trapped in debt, we need to do all we can to see ourselves freed from it. We do this through working and paying the price to be free financially. Walking in humility, we take every financial decision we make seriously and live it out responsibly. Get out of the trap of debt as fast as possible.

It is much easier to get into debt than to get out of debt. Many will help you to get into it, but getting out of it is up to you. Do all you can to eliminate debt. Freedom awaits.

6. Avoid impulsive spending.

There is always a sale. Do not be deceived. Live responsibly. Every time we shop in person or online, our lust button for something flips on. This becomes problematic because what we want, we want now. Impulsive spending can lead to disaster.

At times, one of the wisest things you can do is to delay your decision. Wait for a few days or a week. You may find that you can live without it or you may even forget about it. The human eyes are powerful. Once they lock onto something, it is hard to walk away from it. Refuse to practice impulsive spending.

7. Refuse get-rich-quick schemes.

There is no such thing as getting rich quickly. Refuse to buy into this mentality. Nothing comes without a price. Proverbs 21:5 is a strong encouragement but also a stern warning. It says, "The plans of the diligent certainly lead to profit, but anyone who is reckless certainly becomes poor." We are encouraged that wise and responsible planning will lead us to profit. But we are also warned that recklessness in handling our finances will lead to poverty. Refuse to risk it all by following a sales pitch to get rich quick. There is no such thing.

I hope you will follow the suggestions I have given to you to help you live responsibly through your everyday choices.

The Only Thing Money Can Do for You

Years ago while attending a conference, I heard leadership guru and bestselling author John Maxwell say something along the lines of: *The only thing money can do for you is give you more options.* This was highly impactful in my life.

You see, the less money you have, the fewer options you have. The more money you have, the more options you have.

When we live responsibly, we will have more options before us. When we do not live responsibly, our future becomes limited.

Therefore, hear the heart and feel the passion emerging from the pages of this chapter. Live responsibly.

CHAPTER 15

Live Generously

Generosity is a lifestyle that gives fully and lives openhandedly. Money is necessary to operate in this world. How we choose to handle it and what we choose to do with it will demonstrate how financially fit we really are.

But financial fitness is not determined by the size of our bank accounts. You see, money is a tool, and your worldview determines how you will choose to use it. You will either choose greed or generosity. And it is important to understand that neither greed nor generosity have anything to do with money; each has everything to do with the condition of our hearts.

> Money is a tool, and your worldview determines how you will choose to use it.

What Generosity Is Not

Often, we assume we know what a concept does or does not mean. I do not want to assume anything. What I would like to do is make the meaning of generosity clear.

1. Generosity is not determined by your wealth.

In 2 Corinthians 8, we learn that while the believers in the churches of Macedonia were facing severe affliction, they were also able to experience an abundance of joy. They were living in extreme poverty, yet amazingly, they were overflowing with a wealth of generosity.

Their testimony is remarkable. In spite of their circumstances, they lived out their faith. They lived for the advancement of God's kingdom. They lived generously.

When I read their testimony, I think of so many people I've known through the years who live this way. Facing life against all odds, their gracious attitude emerges.

Generosity like this is not normal. Generosity like this imparts not only monetary support, but gifts of spiritual wealth. Christianity is being lived out by their testimony.

2. Generosity is not determined by how much you give.

How do you measure generosity? When does it become generosity? When you give $50? $500? $1,000? Absolutely not! Generosity is not determined by how much money you give, but by the posture and heart from which you give. Generosity is not determined by giving the first tenth of your entire income. This is the floor for our giving, not the ceiling.

What the Bible Says about Generosity

Second Corinthians 8:3 says, "I can testify that, according to their ability and even beyond their ability, of their own accord, they begged us earnestly for the privilege of sharing in the ministry to the saints." The Bible says their generosity began with giving according to their ability. While their resources were limited, their giving was generous.

This is proportionate giving. This is giving according to their resources. This verse says they gave even beyond their ability. This means they gave beyond their own resources and powers.

This is sacrificial giving because it is beyond their ability or their means to give by their human reasoning. Both proportionate and sacrificial giving was done in this text as an act of their accord or by their will to give. They were not coerced but gave voluntarily and willingly.

In 2 Corinthians 8, we discover the truth that generous giving begins with the willingness of the giver. As God puts it on their heart, they give proportionately and move toward sacrificial giving.

Speaking of the heart, the words of Jesus, which are direct and prophetic, apply to each of us. He said, as recorded in Matthew 6:21, "For where your treasure is, there your heart will be also." Generosity is an issue of the heart. We want to give generously in response to the grace God has given to us. With your life transformed by God's grace, there is nothing that should keep you from giving back to God.

You cannot out-give God. It does not matter how much you give to Him. Shovel out His resources to His Church and His work around the world. His shovel is always bigger than yours.

Generous giving began in the Old Testament. A great example is when the Israelites gave resources for building the Temple.[1] Their willingness to give was indicative that they were giving themselves to the Lord wholeheartedly.

Prior to giving to the Temple, the model of generosity was demonstrated through the giving of God's people to the Tabernacle. While the Temple giving took place in David's day, giving to the Tabernacle was in Moses' day. They gave so generously that the people came to Moses and told him in Exodus 36:5, "'The people are bringing more than is needed for the construction of the work the LORD commanded to be done.'" Moses sent a proclamation throughout the camp in Exodus 36:6, "'Let no man or woman make anything else as an offering for the sanctuary.' So the people stopped."

Both of these illustrations in the Old Testament were marked by outrageous generosity. The people were so captivated by the vision, they gave fully and lived openhandedly.

The heart of generosity was built upon the ancient model of first-tenth giving. While some may choose to minimize or excuse this as irrelevant, I disagree completely. Prior to the Law of Moses, first tenth giving was the beginning step of honoring God with the resources He had entrusted to us. In Genesis 14, over four hundred years prior to the Mosaic Law, Abraham gave one tenth of all he had to God. Abraham was a wealthy man, and this gift must have been significant.

Abraham was returning from a major victory over several kings. Upon returning, he was greeted by Melchizedek, the King of Salem, who is believed by many to have been a revelation of Christ.[2] Immediately upon receiving the blessing from Melchizedek, Abraham called him Sovereign Lord, God Most High. He knew God had handed over his enemies to him. In response to God's miraculous work, Abraham gave to God a tenth of everything he had. This is where tithing or first tenth giving began. This planted seeds of generosity that God has blessed greatly.

One tenth, or first fruits giving, is giving to and honoring God with at least the first ten percent—the best—of everything He has given you.

The Living Bible illustrates this powerfully in its paraphrase of Deuteronomy 14:23. It says, "The purpose of tithing is to teach you always to put God first in your lives." Giving the first tenth is not only an action that shows God is first in your life, it is a realization that the other ninety percent is His also. Remember, God owns everything, and we own absolutely nothing.

The dynamic passage in Malachi 3:10 brings together giving the first tenth and more into the gospel's dimension of generosity. Malachi 3:10 says, "'Bring the full tenth into the storehouse so that there may be food in my house. Test me in this way,' says the Lord of Armies. 'See if I will not open the floodgates of heaven and pour out a blessing for you without measure.'" The tithe tells us the amount of the offering, while first fruits denotes the nature of the gift. The full tenth is a full ten percent of all God has given you in your life. When we give the full tenth, we do it because we love God and believe all that He has given to us is His, not ours. Giving the full tenth is a tangible way of telling God we love Him.

Tithing is never a money issue but a heart issue. It is all about the matter and condition of your heart. I believe that tithing or first fruits giving occurred prior to the Law, under the Law, and now in the age of grace. Jesus tithed.[3] When Jesus discussed tithing with the Pharisees, He encouraged them to continue doing so. I deduce from this that Jesus practiced tithing Himself because He would never encourage others to do what He Himself did not do. The early church understood the nature of generous giving, which I believe is beyond the first-tenth. Paul, when writing to the Corinthians, encouraged them to give from their love for Christ.[4] Grace always fulfills the Law and even more.

Storehouse tithing means you give to the place where God's name dwells. Both Testaments affirm that we should give to a local church to carry out the ministry regionally and globally.[5] The Church is the gathering of people where the name of God is lifted high. Jesus formulated His Church, and it is dwelling globally through the work of hundreds of thousands of local gospel churches. This is where we honor God with our giving of the first tenth and more.

God challenges the people not only to test His plan, but also to follow His plan. When we do this, the windows of heaven open up and pour out upon us blessings that will meet our needs—even if those needs are met in ways we never imagined.

> Generous giving is founded upon the conviction to put God first in your life.

Therefore, generous giving is founded upon the conviction to put God first in your life. With open hands, you willingly give Him your very best, not just the first tenth, but above and beyond because of His work in your life.

When you realize God owns everything and you own absolutely nothing, you live with your hands open, not clinched in a fist. Open hearts and open hands lead to generosity. Closed hearts and closed hands lead to greed.

God wants each of us to live generously. Generosity is a lifestyle that gives fully and lives openhandedly. This leads to living fit financially.

What Generosity Is

Thus far in this chapter, I have shared with you what generosity is not. I have also shared several passages of Scripture that have looked specifically into generosity. I have even taken you back to some of the hallmark passages of the Old Testament that are pivotal to understanding generosity.

Since the first sentence in this chapter, I have defined generosity. I believe generosity is a lifestyle that gives fully and lives openhandedly. When you realize God owns everything and you own absolutely nothing, you live with your hands open, not clinched in a fist.

How does this happen? By understanding even more of what generosity is.

1. Generosity is giving yourself to the Lord.

In 2 Corinthians 8, the people renewed themselves to the Lord. They awakened again to the grace of God they had experienced in their lives. They became willing to do whatever the Lord wanted them to do. They gave themselves to God again.

Generosity begins with giving yourself completely to the Lord. When we dedicate ourselves personally to God in a new and fresh way, generous giving will flow organically from our lives.

How can we not respond to the grace of God with generosity? When we become captivated by His grace and His presence in our lives, we are moved to a new level of surrender to the Lord where we declare, "Whatever you want!"

This is why I have believed for years that giving is a matter of the heart. It is not something we determine because of our assets; it is something we practice because our hearts belong completely to God. We are on our way to living fit financially when we have given ourselves completely to God.

2. Generosity is giving yourself to others.

We need to be over-and-above givers to the Lord, but we also need to be over-and-above givers to people. A generous person looks at people, money, assets, and resources differently because they have given themselves completely to God.

Second Corinthians 8:5 says, "Instead, they gave themselves first to the Lord and then to us by God's will." What a powerful testimony. This should be our testimony. Give your life fully to God and then give yourself freely to others.

3. Generosity is giving money away.

When you have given yourself to God in a fresh way and given yourself to others in a special way, it is easy to give money away.

Generosity is not about money but the condition of your heart. When your heart is right, you live your life openhandedly.

Martin Luther spoke of the need for three conversions: conversion of the heart, conversion of the mind, and conversion of the purse.[6] While spiritual conversion is immediate, sanctification is a process. Luther was right when he stated the sequence of the sanctifying experience of salvation.

I believe that when a person gives God all of their heart and all they have been given, they will discover that God's way is always the best way. I also believe they will discover that, even though it may hurt in the short term, they will never *ultimately* miss any money or assets they give away.

Think about it this way: *Your monthly bank statement is a theological declaration of what you believe about God.* It does not lie. Not just about the money itself, but far more importantly, it tells you about the condition of your heart.

When your heart is fully open to God, your hands follow. You live openhandedly. When your heart becomes closed to the things of God, you live your life grasping and holding on to what you think is yours.

God owns everything and you own absolutely nothing. When you live knowing this, your heart is given to God and you live your life openhandedly. This is generosity. This is why we must choose to live generously.

CHAPTER 16

Live Indelibly

People leave legacies. A legacy cannot be removed. It is a mark that cannot be erased.

An indelible life cannot be removed or erased. This chapter calls upon you to live indelibly. Will you respond to this challenge?

According to the *Merriam-Webster Dictionary*, the word *indelible* describes something "that cannot be removed, washed away or erased."[1]

Placing this unique challenge within this section on living fit financially takes our lives to a new level. When you live wisely, responsibly, and generously relating to money, you have the capacity to live indelibly.

Quite honestly, this should become a BHAG for each one of us. *A BHAG is a Big, Hairy, Audacious Goal.* When a BHAG is reached, major change occurs and a legacy is made.

Why would we not want to live in such a way that our legacy cannot be erased or removed? Why would we not believe we could live indelibly? Why would we not believe God wants to use us to change someone else's life, impact the members of our family for generations, and even become a catalytic force that would make an eternal difference?

I believe all of this is possible with God.

Your Most Important Portfolio

A portfolio is most often mentioned in relationship to money. A person's financial portfolio includes a list of financial assets they hold. If an estate planner is working with you or you are attempting to secure some level of financing, they may request more information than what is known on your basic financial portfolio. You may be asked about your stock portfolio, retirement portfolio, and even your property portfolio. Depending on your age, financial income, and career, each of these may or may not be necessary. Regardless, their goal would be to find out what your entire financial net worth may be.

While someone's financial portfolio is important, is it *the* most important portfolio? Your *life portfolio* is the most important portfolio there is. In this chapter, think about your entire life, not just your finances. Expand your vision and see the possibilities beyond the horizon for all the ways you can determine to live indelibly.

Since people leave legacies, living fit spiritually, physically, relationally, financially, and emotionally is critical. Your life portfolio will not grow if any one of these five areas of your life is unhealthy. The greater your life portfolio is, the more influence your life can have now, in future generations, and in eternity.

> Your life portfolio is the most important portfolio there is.

Identify and Remove the Barriers

Since our goal in this chapter is to live indelibly, we must ask, *What is standing in our way?* When a person or organization desires to grow, part of the process is to take the time to identify and remove the barriers to growth.

We attempt to go out and grow, grow, and grow more, but little to nothing happens. Oftentimes, we get the cart before the horse. We become frustrated and discouraged.

But then, we stop long enough to identify and remove the barriers to our growth. If we have done this accurately, effectively, and in a timely way, growth begins to occur. Therefore, let's get things in the right order now, not later.

I want to identify four barriers to living a life that leaves a legacy that cannot be removed. After identifying the barriers, you can take action to remove them. Then, your entire life portfolio is ready for exponential growth and dynamic legacy impact.

1. An unprioritized life

What are your priorities in life? Do your family and friends know what your priorities are? Does anyone in your workplace know what they are?

I am convinced the more unprioritized your life is, the less impactful it will be. This is why you need to remove the clutter in your life, stop long enough to evaluate who you are and what God wants from your life, and then re-establish your priorities. Your priorities should not be determined by what your preferences are, but what is right biblically. We need to see our priorities as clearly as God does.

Jesus said in Matthew 6:33, "But seek first the kingdom of God and his righteousness, and all these things will be provided for you." Seeking God's kingdom and His righteousness, and the presence and the rule of Jesus Christ in each area of your life, should be the highest priority for Christ-followers. Nothing is greater or higher than the presence, power, and righteousness of Jesus Christ.

Reestablish and then live every area of your life in kingdom priority. I am often asked what our priorities in life ought to be. Let me suggest the following:

- Your personal walk with Jesus Christ daily
- Your family
- Your local church
- Your job and career
- Your recreation

Decision-making is simplified when priorities are established clearly and then lived daily. When you understand what your priorities are, you are ready to remove the huge barrier of living an unprioritized life.

2. An undisciplined life

When you understand what your priorities should be but you are inconsistent in living them out, it shows you are living an undisciplined life. Just as an Olympic athlete works out consistently and by the book, you have to live out your priorities in a disciplined manner each day by God's Book, the Bible!

A lack of discipline leads to inconsistency and a failure to follow through. If this becomes the pattern for most of your life, others will see your walk does not match your talk. As a result, integrity and credibility will be gone. If this happens, you will forfeit the privilege to live indelibly.

Refuse to live an undisciplined life. Take control over your spiritual life, your personal schedule, your physical health, your relationships, and your own emotional health. Living a disciplined life will lead you to make a mark that will ascend your life and legacy for generations and for eternity.

3. A shackled life

Are you living a shackled life that binds you with the chains of your past, relational dysfunction, your health, financial debt, and your own emotional health?

Take the time to identify anything in your life that shackles or binds you. Wherever you are and whatever is binding you, Jesus can set you free. Are you living a shackled life related to any of the following?

- Past—Determine to take it to God and let it go!
- Relationships—Take whatever actions are necessary to establish health in all your relationships.
- Health—Initiate a new commitment to your own health and wellness that starts right where you are, becoming a healthier you.
- Debt—Take definitive actions to eliminate as much debt as possible so that one day, perhaps, you can be debt free.
- Baggage—Clean out any baggage you have emotionally that is holding you back from the life God has for you.

God has no desire for you to live bound or shackled by anything.

The words of Jesus in John 8:32 are appropriate here: "You will know the truth, and the truth will set you free." Remove these chains that shackle you and become all God wills for you to become in your life. Choose freedom.

4. A limited life

Embrace a vision for your future that is unlimited. When all you imagine about yourself and your future is what you can see or what others can see, you are limiting yourself and your future. God has more for you than you can even imagine. Ephesians 3:20 says, "Now to him who is able to do above and beyond all that we ask or think according to the power that works in us." Pursue the above-and-beyond vision and future God has for your life.

It is now time to shed your limited, jaded perspective, and embrace the vision God has for your life. God wills for you to make a mark with your life that no one can erase. Let Him do it!

When any or all of these barriers are taken down, you are able to see and believe God again for ways to live and leave a mark that is indelible. The kind of mark that no one, no problem, and no amount of time can ever erase.

Six Ways You Can Leave an Indelible Mark with Your Life

Since you are determining to identify and remove barriers to living indelibly, I want to share six ways you can do so.

1. Unique godliness

I believe there are certain things you can do to be known for unique characteristics of godliness, not only in this lifetime, but even beyond your death. Not only for now, but even after you are gone.

The Bible says in 1 Timothy 6:6, "But godliness with contentment is great gain." When a person has a unique, godly characteristic, generations to come can be influenced positively.

This is why we could sit around and talk about someone in our family, church, or workplace, and say, "I will never forget her because she was so _____. I wish I could be like her." Godliness with contentment is great gain.

2. Godly children

When you model godliness for your children, you are leaving an indelible mark with your life. This is done in an ongoing manner. As they are growing up in your home, the impact of teaching them to love God is a powerful testimony and legacy.

> The greatest testimony and indelible mark a parent can leave is godly children. They can impact generations.

When we had children in the home, I was asked almost weekly, "Pastor, how can I pray for your children?" For two decades, my answer to these intercessors was always the same. I would ask them to please pray my boys would grow up loving Jesus and loving the church. God answers prayer. Now, my boys are raising their children to do the same.

The greatest testimony and indelible mark a parent can leave is godly children. They can impact generations.

3. Inheritance to your grandchildren

Proverbs 13:22 says, "A good man leaves an inheritance to his grandchildren." When we practice integrity daily, we can leave the inheritance of our integrity to our grandchildren. When we practice faithfulness to our spouse daily, we can leave the inheritance of our faithfulness to our grandchildren. When we practice sound and wise financial principles, we can even leave a financial inheritance to each grandchild.

These inheritances can only be given when we have tamed our tongue, tone, desires, and preferences. As we restrain ourselves along the way of life, this can be a positive, long-term legacy for future generations.

4. Praying for others

We never forget the people who pray for us. I believe I am the recipient of God's multiple blessings upon my life because I have been prayed for continually. I also believe that God does not forget the prayers of His people. As God's people cry out to Him, they can leave an eternal investment into the future of God's work around the world.

I have prayed and fasted numerous times for our nation. I have pleaded with God, especially over the last few years, to revive His Church and awaken our nation spiritually. I still believe God will answer this prayer. I think America will experience the next Great Awakening. People have asked me if I am disappointed this has not yet occurred in our generation. Absolutely not. Even if I die today, I firmly believe God has heard my appeal to Him for this next great movement of His Spirit in America.

Our prayers for other people, our church, and our nation may be answered beyond our lifetime. If so, praying consistently has created great and growing faith in my life.

5. Investing in the next generation

Beyond your children and grandchildren, who in the next generation are you investing in? For the last fifteen years, my soul and eyes light up whenever I am investing in the next generation. It can involve a formal presentation, a message, or even an extensive Q and A.

For example, I deeply cherish being asked to speak at some of our collegiate services on Wednesday nights that will have anywhere from 600 to 1,100 college students present depending on the time of year. The same happens when I speak to a university, student group, and even a room of young adults. I fire up when I invest time with any leader younger than me.

What is it that causes this to happen? I am not sure, but I deeply believe that God wants us to continually invest in the next generation.

6. Leaving money upon your death

If you are in debt upon your death, your family and any other beneficiaries you have will not receive as much as you may have desired. If all debt is gone and wise financial planning has occurred throughout your lifetime, your family and all other beneficiaries will prosper more.

Since I was a child, I have given no less than one tenth of all God has given to me through my local church. For most of our marriage together, Jeana and I have far exceeded that floor for giving. Each year we stand amazed at two things: How much we give away and how much God gives to us. As always, His shovel is bigger than my shovel.

One day when we die, we will leave an inheritance to our children as well as our grandchildren. Additionally, we will leave no less than ten percent of all God has given to us to our local church. Beyond our local church—which is always our priority and I believe God's priority in giving—we will leave other monies for ministry. We do this now and we will do it when we die.

I would like to encourage every follower of Jesus Christ to, upon their death, leave no less than ten percent of their entire estate to their church. Some may desire to leave a far greater percentage. *I believe we should die in the same way we lived—honoring God financially with all He has entrusted to us through our local church!*

It may be unwise to leave sums of money too large from your estate to your children if they do not honor God with their life and choices. You are a steward even in your death, and you need to shepherd your estate with wisdom by following godly counsel from God's Word. Use your estate to invest into the kingdom of

God more than ever before! This can be a tremendous testimony to your children.

In considering these six ways you can leave an indelible mark with your life, I want to quote from bestselling author and leadership equipper John Maxwell. In the foreword for *The Eternity Portfolio*, Maxwell writes these stirring words:

> What would happen if we saw giving as a way of investing? If we gave our giving "portfolio" the same attention we give our retirement portfolio? What would happen if we stopped asking, "How much do I have to give?" and start asking, "How much can I invest in eternity by giving?" How would our lives change if we became aware of the rewards of faithfully investing our resources?[2]

What would happen if you implemented John's stirring challenge? It would change your life and your attitude. It would also greatly impact eternity.

Begin to invest in eternity now. Do not wait until your death. But when your death occurs and your estate is settled, make sure you have invested in eternity.

This is just one of the many ways, but a very significant way for you to leave a mark with your life that no one will ever erase or remove. Live indelibly.

SECTION 5

Living Fit Emotionally

CHAPTER 17

Live Watchfully

Living Fit is a conversation created to help you recognize, read, and monitor the different gauges in your life. Just as in your car, gauges are instruments that measure significant markers.

Early one morning while I was working on this manuscript, Jeana went to a class she regularly attends at the fitness center. As she was almost there, she called to tell me the fuel gauge on her car said she had only twenty-seven miles of fuel left in the tank, and had not realized this before leaving the house. As you know, this projection all depends on if the gauge is reading accurately and the way you drive the car. This was not a healthy situation to be in, but the fitness club is located within seven minutes of our home.

Since she was headed to the gym, all Jeana had with her was her driver's license, and no cash. She decided that since she was in a rush with early appointments, she would just drive home after her class and deal with the fuel issue later.

My plan was to write in my home office most of the day, so after she returned home, I told her to take my vehicle and I would take care of putting fuel in her vehicle later. I was busy writing, and I ended up working from home the entire day.

The next day, she reminded me about her vehicle, and that she needed fuel in her car immediately. So, as we were on our way to run an errand together, all based upon what the gauge had informed us, the first thing we did was go two miles from our home to fill her car with fuel. Relief occurred when the gauge read full.

If Jeana had ignored the gauge completely, acting like it was not important, she would have ended up on the side of the interstate in a needful and dangerous situation. But Jeana recognized what the gauge was telling her, read it accurately, monitored its progress, and acted accordingly.

Gauges are there for a reason. They communicate helpful and potentially life-saving messages, giving information you and I need to know. As you create the discipline to check the gauges in your life, you need to have the discernment to act wisely upon what they inform you about your life.

Where You Are Now

Our conversation has taught you to recognize several gauges in your life, relating to your spiritual, physical, relational, and financial health. Now you are equipped to recognize each one of these gauges, learn everything you can about them, monitor them consistently, and do whatever is necessary to move each one to the most positive reading possible at this time in your life. The goal is not personal perfection, but personal progress. Where are you now?

> The goal is not personal perfection, but personal progress. Where are you now?

In the first four sections of the book, I have shared with you about four specific gauges in your personal life. These are your:

- Spiritual gauge
- Physical gauge
- Relational gauge
- Financial gauge

The vision for *Living Fit* is to help you make your life count by pursuing a healthy you. Every person is different and uniquely created by God, but we are all called to pursue spiritual, physical, relational, and financial fitness. Where are you with each one of these? What is each gauge telling you about your personal life?

Since your entire life is connected and not compartmentalized, each one of these instruments is connected to the others. My personal conviction is this: *As your spiritual life goes, so goes the rest of your life.* In other words, your spiritual life is the center of who you are and is the common and interconnected force in your entire life.

As we introduce the fifth and final gauge that is necessary to recognize, read, monitor, and act upon, it is imperative for us to have a common understanding. Our common understanding is that whatever is happening in your life—spiritually, physically, relationally, and financially—will lead to what is going on in this fifth area of your life. If any of these first four areas are suffering, I assure you, living fit emotionally will be far more difficult.

This fifth section will challenge you and continue the conversation by focusing on living fit emotionally. In this section, I will encourage you to:

- Live Watchfully
- Live Respectfully
- Live Gratefully
- Live Wholly

This section will be somewhat different from the others because it relies on the previous work done in the process of our calling to be fit.

Remember, *the process always precedes the product*. In this process of pursuing a healthy you, it will be extremely challenging for you to become healthy emotionally if you are not fit spiritually, physically, relationally, and financially. Your emotional health, whether it is good, inconsistent, or poor, is determined mostly by the condition of these other four areas of your life. Therein, the number one need at this point in the journey to fitness is to:

Live Watchfully

The body God has given each of us is quite amazing. Any level of health we have is a blessing from Him.

There are times a person's body enters into a critical state of health. Whether it is following a surgical procedure or the experience of trauma, or a serious illness, their life hangs in the balance. Within hours or a few days, the family is informed that all signs point to their body beginning to shut down, and in all probability, impending death. The medical professionals explain the process, showing the connectedness of the body, how one thing has led to another, and why the end is now near.

These professionals know this for two reasons. First, they have been watchful since the beginning of what has caused this issue in the body. Second, the instruments they used with the patient could tell them things they could not see with their eyes.

Just as it is important for medical professionals to be watchful with patients who are in critical condition, it is important for you to be watchful over your entire life. It is important for you to sense where you are, but more importantly, to know where you are.

This requires you to live watchfully!

Watch Over Your Life

Watch what is going on around you. Watch what is going on in you. Watch what all the gauges are telling you about your life.

In the Scripture, we are instructed to watch over our life and all God gives to us.[1] Our future way in life and even the preservation of our life can depend on our intentionality, discipline, and watchfulness.

The Bible calls upon the watchman to watch over the city at night while others sleep.[2] The Bible also calls upon spiritual watchmen to watch over the people of God in prayer continually.[3] It also calls each person to watch out for people around them.[4] We are even told to watch for the Lord's soon return.[5]

There is another way we see this word *watch* used in the Scripture, depending on the translation. We are called upon to watch over our own life, to avoid evil, and to protect our life.

Proverbs 16:17 says, "The highway of the upright avoids evil; the one who guards his way protects his life." If you will keep your life going on the right highway, you will avoid evil or any detour from the road that God wants you to travel. Then the Scripture says that as you guard or watch over your own life effectively, you will protect or keep your life from trouble in the future.

The word translated here as *guard* is the Hebrew word *nat sar*, meaning to guard, watch over, or keep watch over your life so you can observe it properly, and save your life.[6]

I find it interesting how various translations and paraphrases communicate the heart of the verse. Notice these examples from Proverbs 16:17.

- "The highway of the upright is to depart from evil; He who keeps his way preserves his soul." (NKJV)
- "The highway of the upright turns aside from evil; whoever guards his way preserves his life." (ESV)

- "The highway of the upright is to depart from evil: he that keepeth his way preserveth his soul." (KJV)
- "The highway of the upright is to depart from evil; He who watches his way preserves his life." (NASB)
- "The path of the godly leads away from evil; he who follows that path is safe." (TLB)
- "The road of right living bypasses evil; watch your step and save your life." (*The Message*)

Each of these offers a nuanced perspective, but the translations and interpretations are consistent. They all relate to guarding, watching, or keeping. We are called to carefully watch over our lives.

How You Watch Will Determine If You Are Living Fit Emotionally

What is going on around you will, many times, bring out what is really in you. This can be quite revealing. When the wheels of your life start to fall off, your emotional gauge begins to reflect it.

I remember hearing evangelist and revivalist Manley Beasley Sr. speak about this during my college years. Brother Manley, as everyone called him then, used to use a lemon as an illustration. He would ask what would come out of a lemon if you squeezed it. Inevitably, someone from the audience would respond with, "Lemon juice." Brother Manley would ultimately disagree with the assessment of the audience. He would ask how they knew someone hadn't injected something else into the lemon with a syringe. Each person in the audience would shake their head in agreement and smile. Then, Brother Manley would ask the question again,

> When the wheels of your life start to fall off, your emotional gauge begins to reflect it.

but go on to give the answer. Everyone in the audience was drawn into his illustration, yearning to know what would come from the lemon. He would smile and say that when you squeeze a lemon, what comes out of it is what's inside it.

Then Brother Manley would use this illustration to tell you the same thing about your life and my life. When the pressures of life come and we are squeezed, whatever is in us will come out. Sometimes it is frustration, other times it is anger, every now and then it is irritation. Not nearly often enough is it Jesus.

Most often, negativity comes out of us for one reason: we are failing to watch over the gauges of our life. Watchfulness will create orderliness that will bring godliness into our lives more consistently.

Two Actions to Take to Watch over Your Life

Here are two actions to take to watch over your life effectively:

Action 1: Watch your gauges consistently.

Recognize, read, monitor, and act upon what each of the five gauges of your life are registering. Measure consistently to see whether you are living fit spiritually, physically, relationally, financially, and emotionally.

Action 2: Watch your steps daily.

What you do each moment, every day, in these five areas of your life will determine your overall level of fitness. Connectedness exists between each of these areas. It is essential to keep watch over not just each one, but all of them together, because this will determine how healthy you really are. The only antidote to this is to watch your steps daily.

Therefore, a key to living fit is to live watchfully.

CHAPTER 18

Live Respectfully

Respecting where you are emotionally and respecting where others are emotionally will lead you to experience meaningful relationships. This furthers the importance of reading your own life gauges consistently. Then, you will be more equipped to understand where other people may be in their own life journey. When this occurs, your personal relationships will become more meaningful.

Pursuing a healthy you is a high and worthy goal. Different than what most people think, this is an arduous task. It takes personal sacrifice and time. Due to the magnitude, I just do not see it happening without a major spiritual intervention by God. This is why your spiritual life is so important. It cannot be minimized, nor should it be. This vision of a healthy you can only happen with and by God's power.

While you pursue this quest, the demonic forces of hell will fight you all the way. Satan will do all he can to lead you toward how he wants you to see things, rather than seeing things the way God says they are. Life is an ongoing battle that is serious and necessary. It does not get easier. In fact, it gets more fierce than ever before because so much is at stake.

This is why the apostle Paul told the church at Ephesus the words recorded in Ephesians 6:11, "Put on the full armor of God so that you can stand against the schemes of the devil." The next series of verses speaks of each piece of the armor and its role in the life of the Christ follower.

Each morning, I put on the armor of God in prayer, piece-by-piece. Not only for myself, but also for the entire Floyd Team comprised of Jeana and me, our two sons, our daughters-in-law, and our grandchildren. You see, I learned a long time ago that Satan is trying to steal, kill, and destroy our lives. If I ignore it, my family becomes open prey for him. This is one of the major reasons I have called out to God in prayer each morning. The necessity is laid upon me.

All this is so important because we fight not only against Satan and his demonic forces, but we also have an ongoing war with our own flesh. Our own flesh does not accommodate a passion for Christ, nor does it adjust to it. The apostle Paul wrote about this type of warfare with the church at Galatia in Galatians 5:16–17, "I say then, walk by the Spirit and you will certainly not carry out the desire of the flesh. For the flesh desires what is against the Spirit, and the Spirit desires what is against the flesh; these are opposed to each other, so that you don't do what you want." It is clear that we cannot win our own personal battle against our flesh without the intervention of God's Spirit. This is serious warfare that demands the best from us.

Herein lies the challenge of having an authentic self-awareness in our conversation about becoming and living fit spiritually, physically, relationally, financially, and emotionally. The big question I believe we need to answer is: How do you live respectfully? How do you come to the point of respecting where you are emotionally and respecting where others are emotionally? Is this really what it means to have meaningful relationships?

I believe answering the first question effectively answers the rest of them. So, how do you live respectfully? I believe the answer involves three important practices in your life.

> The big question I believe we need to answer is: How do you live respectfully?

Accept Yourself

Accepting yourself for who you are in Christ and where you are in your life is critical to experiencing peace within and meaningful relationships with others. My personal belief is that accepting yourself usually begins to be a struggle in childhood, then deepens greatly in your teenage years, and is seemingly continuous through your adult years.

This is a challenge for each person through every stage of life. Most of the time, we settle into a comfort zone and stay there. If we don't, we feel we are at risk for personal disappointment and hurt.

Years ago, God began to help me work through this personally. Through the reading and studying of the Bible, one day the Lord opened my eyes to this issue. It came through reading Romans 15:7, "Therefore accept one another, just as Christ also accepted you, to the glory of God." This call to accept one another means you are taking another by the hand, opening your heart, and drawing them into your life.

The strong appeal in this passage is to accept one another even as Christ accepted us. As the Messiah, he entered this world as a Jew, but His life and vision were far bigger than just his own ethnic people—He came for the nations. So the appeal, relating to others in your life now or others you will meet, is to always accept them because God has accepted you in Christ.

I was enlightened by the Spirit to understand that since Christ accepted me and I am to accept others, surely I must also accept myself. This was verified through my growing faith and the deepening knowledge of the Word of God. The reason we struggle so much with accepting ourselves is because we have forgotten Jesus accepted us at salvation and still does today through sanctification. Since Jesus accepts me, I must be willing to accept myself.

Do you accept yourself? Do you accept all your good, all your challenges, and even all your failures? Do you accept yourself for who you are as a person and where you are in your life presently?

I believe the key to this is having what I call an authentic self-awareness. Let's discuss this further.

Authentic Self-Awareness

The word *authentic* is thrown around so much on the Internet today that I usually run from even using it. Yet, I will use it today because I think this is the right word.

Authentic means what is real, actual, or true.[1] It is not something copied or done to conform to what one perceives someone else wants.

Do you have an authentic self-awareness? Do you look at yourself honestly and realistically?

Five Observations About Authentic Self-Awareness

I want to share five observations about authentic self-awareness.

1. Authentic self-awareness is an increasing challenge. While authenticity is a buzzword used by so many people today, it is a challenge to have a clear and honest picture about who you really are. Talking about authenticity does not mean authenticity is taking place. With the barrage of information you face each day due to the ubiquity of social media, truth about anything—including yourself—is difficult to evaluate.

Growing older does not guarantee you will have any more clarity about yourself. In fact, it may cloud your view even more. With age, your life changes, your body changes, and at times, even your desires change. You may begin to delude yourself, which is not helpful for anyone.

Sometimes success adds to the increasing challenge of authentic self-awareness. When people say things about you in a public manner, good or bad, it makes it more difficult to see yourself in a healthy way. Periodically, I challenge people to remember that when you believe everything good people say about you, then you will also have to believe everything bad they say about you. It's best to be cautious in our response to both.

This is why it is an increasing challenge to practice authentic self-awareness.

2. Authentic self-awareness is a perilous quest. Scripture warns us to not deceive ourselves.[2] This means self-deception does occur, and the power of imagining ourselves to be something we are not is an ongoing threat for each of us. It also means that we often miscalculate who we are through false reasoning and delusion. Authentic self-awareness is a perilous quest, because deception lies around every corner.

Be careful. Peer pressure can often press in on you personally, tempting you to pretend to be something you really are not. Personal pride enters in, and all of a sudden, you become blind about who you are and what you do well. This leads to discontentment. Soon after, you take another job and within months, realize you are not in your sweet spot.

People telling you what you ought to be doing with your life will lead you to deceiving yourself. Be careful. Be wise. Be discerning. Authentic self-awareness is important. Rest in who God made you to be.

3. Authentic self-awareness is a spiritual imperative.
Evaluate yourself continually. Make this a regular part of your spiritual journey. Appeal for God's help. Ask the Holy Spirit to show you who you really are.

As you read the Bible, always pay close attention to any counsel about who you are in Christ. You are not who you think you are, nor who others believe you are; you are who God says you are. From this point of biblical authority, reflect upon who God has made you to be and gifted you to be. You are a work in progress to the glory of God.

> You are not who you think you are, nor who others believe you are; you are who God says you are.

4. Authentic self-awareness is a personal wake-up call. If and when God shows you any variance to who you think you are versus the reality of who you are, let it serve as a personal wake-up call. It should call you to ask Him for His intervention in revealing the truth about yourself to you.

If this happens, deal with it spiritually. Confess it to God and receive His forgiveness. Then, go forward being filled with and walking in the Spirit. Deal with it practically. Adjust your life and desires to it. Refuse to be coerced into trying to be someone God has not really made you to be.

5. Authentic self-awareness is a healthy respect for who you are and where you are in your life. God made you special. There is no one else like you. Having a healthy respect for yourself is important. You do not have to succumb to the pressure of other people. Living respectfully is accepting yourself.

This involves accepting who you are, but it also involves accepting where you are. Where you are is another plea to see yourself through your life gauges. There are times when you may not be fit in one or more of these areas: spiritual, physical, relational, financial, or emotional. Accept yourself enough that you are willing to be honest about each of these areas.

Respecting where you are in each of these areas will give you some insights into being all God wants you to be. Therefore, reflect, be honest, and take action when you understand more about yourself.

Accept Others

Living respectfully involves both accepting yourself and accepting others. I am convinced that one of the reasons we struggle at times accepting other people is we have never accepted ourselves.

Even Jesus came to His own people and they did not receive Him. John 1:11 says, "He came to his own, and his own people did not receive him." They had a very unhealthy view of themselves, and this is why Jesus told them they were blind to who He was and is—the Messiah. Because they didn't accept the reality of who they were—sinners in need of a Savior—they couldn't accept the reality that He had come to save them. John 1:12 says, "But to all who did receive him, he gave them the right to be children of God, to those who believe in his name."

Here is what must happen if we are going to live respectfully.

We need to receive Christ personally. When we realize that because of what Christ did on the cross, He has accepted us; and we can begin to accept ourselves and others.

When you see other people through the five life gauges in this book, you are able to discern where they are more accurately, and you are ready to enter into a more meaningful relationship with them. This equips you to meet their needs much more effectively. Love is meeting needs.

Act Wisely

Most of this chapter has been spent talking about accepting yourself. I have done this intentionally because this is such a great challenge. Please understand, when you accept yourself, you are able to then accept others more effectively. From this position of accepting yourself and accepting others, act wisely.

Do not be reckless with your words within any given situation.

The secret to acting wisely is not in reacting to others and to situations impulsively, but responding wisely.

You cannot control other people. You cannot control situations and circumstances. You can control only one thing—your response to them.

This is why you need to act wisely.

Refuse to cast judgment too quickly. Ask God to give you spiritual discernment about people and where they are as well as their situations or circumstances. Always remember that arrogance divides people, but respect honors people.

What is in you will come out when the pressure is on in your life. Emotional outbursts and exaggerations are always a signal there is a deeper issue going on. Living fit emotionally is a tremendous challenge for every person.

But here is what I do know about living fit emotionally. It is necessary for me to live watchfully by always monitoring the gauges of my life and what is going on within me. Then, I need to live respectfully by receiving myself for who God has made me to be and what He has me doing right now. Only then am I ready to receive others for who they are and what God has made them to be. Interestingly, when I do this well, my relationships are much more meaningful and effective.

Therefore, live respectfully.

CHAPTER 19

Live Gratefully

In September of my junior year in college, I began serving as a local church pastor. Jeana and I would be married that December. Each weekend, I drove sixty-five miles each way to serve as pastor of this church in a town of three hundred people.

Looking back, I now know the truth. They needed a pianist. Jeana was about to graduate with a degree in music education, and piano was her concentration. She was a much better pianist than I was a preacher. In all reality, they probably tolerated me as their pastor while they loved Jeana as their pianist. Beginning three months prior to our marriage, we would go and minister to those sweet and grateful people.

When I fast forward to today, I see a vast difference in serving people. There is a major shift in the attitude of people today compared to people then. I believe I know what it is.

Later, when I began serving larger churches, I was able to have staff team members who would help me bear the load of my responsibilities. Today, in our multi-campus church, our staff team is very large. For the last decade or so, I have noticed this same decline in the attitude of staff members. At first, I could not figure it out. But I now know what it is.

Over a decade ago, when one of our team members believed God had called them to another ministry, before they left, they would usually set up a time for us to spend together. They would come to my office or we would eat lunch together casually. They would begin by telling me how grateful they were for their time here and why they were grateful. Then, they would humbly say something like this: *"Pastor, before I left, I not only wanted to come in and say thank you, but I want you to be honest with me. How can I become a better person and a more effective leader?"* Over a decade ago, it would have been rare if this kind of conversation did not take place before we sent them out to their next ministry with our blessing.

There are times now when a staff member will not share their appreciation for their time on staff, or even think to ask for advice on how they might improve themselves. Why is this?

I believe the decline in attitude can be attributed to *ingratitude.* The spirit of ungratefulness is a warning sign of being emotionally unhealthy. Ungratefulness is not God's will and is, in fact, completely opposite of God's will for our lives.

> When gratitude is your attitude, you are on your way to living fit emotionally.

An ungrateful person repels other people. Their ingratitude is a walking billboard of their unhealthy emotional condition. Their relationships are usually shallow and their influence is limited.

Conversely, when gratitude is your attitude, you are on your way to living fit emotionally. A grateful person is endearing to other people. There is something special and attractive about a person who overflows with gratitude.

Which one of these attitudes represents your life most of the time?

Is it gratitude or ingratitude?

If you want a truthful answer, ask a few people you work with daily. Ask your spouse and your family. What would they say?

This degeneration in attitude across America is highly concerning to me. When the people that fill the churches across our land and even the leaders who serve these churches are known for their ingratitude, we are in a downward spiral. Who do we think we are when we are ungrateful? Do we really think this attitude is what the Lord wills for us? I pray not!

God's Will for You and Your Attitude

Have you ever considered what God's will is for you and your attitude? This is a worthy consideration and a question that deserves to be answered.

The answer is found in the Bible. When the Bible speaks, God speaks. What is He saying to us?

First Thessalonians 5:18 says, "Give thanks in everything; for this is God's will for you in Christ Jesus." I believe this is very clear. God wants us to give thanks and overflow with gratitude. Giving thanks is being grateful and expressing this gratitude personally, privately, and publicly.

Immediately before this verse calling us to live out God's will with gratitude and thankfulness for all things, God says in 1 Thessalonians 5:16-17, "Rejoice always, pray constantly." This is what sets up the clear declaration of God's will for us in verse 18.

- Rejoice always.
- Pray constantly.
- Give thanks in everything.

While these verses are brief, they are profound.

Joy is always appropriate in the life of a Christian. Praying consistently and regularly should represent our lives daily. When joy is present and prayer is ongoing, gratitude will always be overflowing.

Christians frequently discuss what it takes to discover God's will. Sermons are preached about it, lessons are taught on it, and books exist by the volumes about it. When we talk about this topic, we tend to focus on the things that are unclear; but there are certain things that the Bible makes more than clear! One of the most glaring opportunities related to God's will is living a grateful and thankful life. The attitude of gratitude is endearing, attractive, and even contagious! When you are around someone who exudes gratitude, it is much more difficult to fall into the negativity that is so prevalent in the world today.

God wants you to live fit! He wants you to live fit spiritually, physically, relationally, financially, and emotionally. Our emotions most often represent how we are doing in the previous four life gauges. But when it comes to an attitude of ingratitude, this is certainly not God's will.

It is past time that we get ourselves in shape regarding our attitude. God's will for you and your attitude is to live with a grateful heart, overflowing with thankfulness to God and others daily. We are blessed and should declare how blessed we are to a world that desperately needs Christ.

We need to be alert and make sure we do not fall prey to this epidemic of ingratitude that is occurring across the world. If we are even close to falling away from God's will, I believe some warning signs will be going off in us and around us. If they are, it shows we are emotionally unhealthy.

Six Warning Signs of Being Emotionally Unhealthy

There is a downward slope occurring that is undeniable. This descent should concern each of us personally. Notice this downward trend that I believe begins with being ungrateful:

Warning Sign 1: Ingratitude

This downward trend all begins with ingratitude. When you live without a grateful heart daily, you are on the brink of entering into a downward spiral. The inability to say thank you is like a plague. It is a disease that takes away life.

When we are not willing to live grateful lives before others, it is indicative we are not grateful to God. Times of prayer and times in your daily life need to exist when nothing more than thanksgiving flows from your heart, giving thanks to God for everything.

When ingratitude exists in your life, you are near falling off a cliff that is often impossible to find your way back up again. Ingratitude is the opposite of the will of God for your life. God wants you to be thankful, not unthankful. God wants you overflowing with gratitude, not ingratitude.

When you enter a season of ingratitude, it is a warning sign that you are emotionally unhealthy. You need to stop where you are and talk to God. Ask Him to help you deal with your problem immediately. Leave your feelings behind, rising up from the ashes of ingratitude with a grateful heart. When you do, you are entering the will of God. If you choose not to do so, get ready. The following will occur in your life.

Warning Sign 2: Entitlement

The moment you begin thinking you are entitled to certain things, you are entering into dangerous territory. When ingratitude is tolerated in your life, soon you will slide down the slippery slope into an entitlement mentality.

This is so evident in our nation today. People think they are entitled to certain things and the government owes them. The same is true about the Church. People think they are entitled to certain things and the Church owes them. This entitlement mentality goes back to people's view of God. People think God owes them. Let me set the record straight. God owes us nothing. He has already given us everything through His Son and His death on the cross for us. The blessings from the heavenly Father are great and are innumerable; they are far beyond what we could even hope or imagine.

Ingratitude leads downward to entitlement. Where does entitlement lead?

Warning Sign 3: Discontentedness

Contentedness is emotionally constructive. Discontentedness is emotionally destructive. The more content you are, the more grateful you are. Sadly, ingratitude leads to feeling entitled, and this leads to falling into a land of discontentedness.

> The more content you are, the more grateful you are.

We see discontent people all the time. Discontent over the way they look. Discontent over where they live and what they drive. Discontent with their job, having convinced themselves they are entitled to more.

Discontentedness points backward to one glaring reality: an ungrateful heart. Ingratitude always leads to discontentedness.

Warning Sign 4: Skepticism

Continually doubting the truth is not a noble characteristic. This is skepticism. Ingratitude leads to entitlement, entitlement leads to discontentedness, and discontentedness leads to skepticism.

It doesn't matter which newscast, commentary, or editorial you turn to, skepticism is ruling the American mind-set. Skepticism leads you to doubt what the truth really is. This ongoing suspicion is very disheartening.

People hold their skepticism up like a badge of honor, as if they were more enlightened or informed than others. It is, in reality, a badge with one word on it: *Ungrateful!* An ungrateful life will sooner or later fill the rest of life with skepticism. I believe it is nauseating and very unbecoming.

Warning Sign 5: Criticism

Criticism abounds across the American culture. People are critical of our nation, her military, and her leaders. People are even critical of our flag and what it stands for nationally and internationally. People are critical of their best friends and their own family members. People are even critical of the Bible and the Church.

Do you criticize constantly? Is sarcasm, which is nothing more than backhanded criticism, always near your lips? Being critical of other people and leaders of organizations and governments is nothing to be proud of.

A spirit of criticism finds its root in one place: ingratitude! Living an ungrateful life eventually leads to having a critical spirit. When you think you are the only one who is ever right, you are living in deception.

Warning Sign 6: Cynicism

Cynicism is a sneering disbelief in people, their words, and their motives.

This sounds like every evening news and cable news show on television. What a sad commentary on our culture today.

This doesn't just exist in media and politics, but also in American business, education, entertainment, and law. Creating disbelief and casting continual suspicion is highly disturbing, and limits the level of success in our nation.

Even more sadly, cynicism exists in the Church. Quite honestly, I see it more among church leaders and denominational leaders than I see it in members of the Church. Dissecting every word someone says and acting like a theological police force toward other people is pride and arrogance. What a poor testimony before the world.

Just think, it all begins with disobedience to God's will. God's will is for each one of us to give thanks in everything. When we do not, the downward spiral begins:

- Ingratitude
- Entitlement
- Discontentedness
- Skepticism
- Criticism
- Cynicism

These are warning signs that show us we are emotionally unhealthy. The alarm is going off in our lives. We must control this. It is not right. It is not God's will.

We must return to having hearts that are overflowing with gratitude. Gratitude to God for all He has done. Gratitude to others for what they have done for us. Gratitude that still values two of the most powerful words in the English language: "Thank you!" Gratitude that still values the power of a handwritten note to someone. Yes, I am talking about the kind of gratitude that is humble before God and others, endearing to everyone, and even contagious among all.

If you want to set your life, leadership, commitment, and legacy apart, here is the way to do it in today's world: *Give thanks in everything; for this is God's will for you in Christ Jesus* (1 Thess. 5:18).

Live gratefully.

CHAPTER 20

Live Wholly

God desires for you to live a complete and full life in every way. This can only happen when you live wholly.

Living a whole life is rarely discussed, especially from a biblical worldview. Secular self-help books that cast a vision for people to live a full life abound. I am grateful for their vision and desire to help people live up to their potential, even though many of them take an ungodly approach to the way they believe it needs to be achieved.

Christian leaders often run from this topic. They fear being linked to the secular self-help world, or being associated with groups that may be perceived as not biblically and theologically sound. While we need to always use wisdom in the choices we make, we should never fear sharing what God says about all areas of life. Nor should we shy away from calling people to live a whole life.

But in all reality, many in the Christian world do not want to talk about living a whole life because it calls them to accountability in some of the areas of life they have never taken very seriously. For example . . .

- When was the last time you heard the pastor of your church challenge you in your personal spiritual life? Has he called you to do something daring and courageous you have never done before in order to grow in your faith?
- When is the last time you heard the pastor in your church challenge you to get your act together regarding your personal health and wellness?
- When is the last time you heard the pastor in your church challenge you to take the needed actions with God to get your relationship right with Him and restore all relationships in your life that are broken?
- When is the last time you heard the pastor in your church challenge you to get yourself together financially, calling you boldly to honor God with at least the first tenth of all you have and more, to begin to make wise financial decisions regarding budgeting, spending, saving, investing, and eliminating debt?
- When is the last time you heard a pastor in your church challenge you to evaluate your own emotional health and well-being?
- When is the last time you heard a pastor in your church challenge you to see your whole life comprised of the spiritual, physical, relational, financial, and emotional as one, complete, and whole life that God wants to set in order and synergize for His glory and honor?

These questions are not about what your pastor or church is or is not doing. They are simply questions to illustrate how spiritual leaders rarely deal with matters like this specifically, much less as the whole. If your pastor does, he is a champion, and a rare commodity.

In the typical church, you will rarely be challenged personally and boldly about your own spiritual growth. You will never be challenged about your own physical health and well-being. Rarely will a pastor call you to get your life right with God and take all actions necessary to restore all broken relationships. As to financial issues, other than maybe a financial stewardship sermon about giving once every few years, most leaders never talk about the basics like debt or budgeting. When it comes to emotional well-being, this may be acknowledged some by leaders, even though probably done more indirectly. It is even more rare for a spiritual leader to address your whole life being comprised of the spiritual, physical, relational, financial, and emotional as one life to be used for God's glory.

I am so passionate about this because I am convinced that God really desires for you to live a complete and full life in every way. Without a doubt, this can only happen when you live wholly. Is this even possible?

God's Possibility for You

I believe God has so much more for us than we ever even imagine. At times, I believe we settle for much less of a life than God intends because we fail to see that He wants something greater for each of us.

As a parent and grandparent, I plead with God daily for my children and their families. When our two boys were growing up, I wanted the very best for them and did everything I could to make it happen. I want this for their children today. Even though I do not have direct oversight of a child or grandchild, I still yearn for them to each receive the best and fulfill their God-given capacity in life.

If I, even though limited as a human being, so desire this for the members of my family, how much more does God desire it for His children? He wants us to reach the highest capacity He created us to experience on this earth (John 10:10). He loves us, is for us, and is working all things together for our good (Rom. 8:28).[1]

Here is God's possibility for you and your future. I want to look deeper into Ephesians 3:20. It says, "Now to him who is able to do above and beyond all that we ask or think according to the power that works in us."

What does all this mean? The apostle Paul was overwhelmed with the grace of God in his life. After expressing in humility that he was the least of all the saints, he was consumed with preaching the light of the gospel to everyone. From the powerful platform of prayer where he declared he had bold and confident access to the Father, he saw every adversity in his life as a way to bring glory to God.

This is why he bowed on his knees in prayer, calling out to God to give him strength by the power of the Holy Spirit. Paul yearned to abound in the love of God and to understand this love as much as possible. His great passion was to experience the fullness of God.

It was within this biblical context and flow of testimony that Paul broke forth with the robust faith and vision of Ephesians 3:20. This life is possible only when we are humble before God, living by God's power, and abounding in God's love. When we are sold out to God completely, Ephesians 3:20 is possible for each of us to live out daily. Please understand that God has so much more for you than you have ever imagined or comprehended. Do not limit the life that God has for you.

> God has so much more for you than you have ever imagined or comprehended. Do not limit the life that God has for you.

The more robust our devotion to Him, the more robust our vision to see it come to pass occurs. Ephesians 3:20 reminds us that our God is more than capable to do something that is extraordinary, as well as over and above in and through our lives! His "beyond life" for us is "more than more" than we have ever imagined or comprehended. It is even more than we have ever called out to God for in prayer or even considered for our life. How is this all possible? It is only possible to the level that God's power, might, and resources operate within and through us. All for the purpose of bringing God glory and extending His glory to every corner of this universe. This is why he closes this doxology with the words recorded in Ephesians 3:21, "to him be glory in the church and in Christ Jesus to all generations, forever and ever. Amen."

All of this is God's possibility for you. Ephesians 3:20 is God's vision for your life and future. It applies to each segment of your life. This is why I believe it is more than possible for us to live wholly.

How to Live Wholly

Ephesians 3:20 gives us a robust vision to live wholly. How can this be done practically? Live out these three actions.

Action 1: Live with purpose.

I shared extensively about purpose in chapter 3. While I have previously stated its importance, I believe I would be remiss not to mention it briefly again. Living with purpose is critical in order to live wholly.

Knowing God is at work in your life and has purposed you to live for His glory, always remember that God is for you. He is so much for you that He has given you a purpose for your life. Yes, with great conviction and certainty, I believe God has a purpose for your life.

Do not meander through life, chasing one hundred things. Chase after God and His purpose for your life. Pursue His purpose with all your heart. When you face an obstacle or setback, push through it, knowing that nothing can hinder God's purpose for your life. Then, give your life, vision, and future to serving God's purpose in your generation.

God is for you, and Ephesians 3:21 says He wants His glory extended to all generations! Just think, He wants to use you to do it.

Living wholly begins with living your life with purpose.

Action 2: Live your life connecting.

Stop believing that everything in life needs to revolve around you. Stop believing that you do not need other people. You may go faster at times in your life when you go alone, but you will never go farther. How can we ever live wholly if we do not live connecting?

This is why I gave the entire eleventh chapter to the subject of connecting. It cannot be emphasized enough in our narcissistic culture. We need to live connecting.

We need to connect with God daily. I am not talking about checking it off a daily to-do list, but really connecting with God. Just this past Sunday, a man in his eighties walked up to me, one of our church's brightest stars. He asked, "Pastor Ronnie, do you remember when you started challenging our church in 1991 about reading the One Year Bible through annually?" I told him I did. He then told me that each of these years, he had read the Bible through and testified to its impact upon him. His connecting with God through God's Word transformed his life.

We need to connect with the church and with other people. Through the experience of engaging in the local church weekly, our lives can go upward. Dynamic worship moments, small group Bible Study, and serving with others to advance the gospel in our communities and beyond can impact our lives greatly. Living my life on mission with God is much more effective when I know there are friends and fellow soldiers who are taking the name of Jesus with them wherever they go around the world.

Living wholly begins with living your life with purpose. Living wholly progresses your life forward when you live your life connecting.

Action 3: Live up to your capacity.

I believe God desires for you to live your life to reach your capacity. This will depend on you becoming fit in your life. Living fit does not just happen. Living fit can only occur through great intentionality and a commitment to living a more disciplined life.

You cannot reach your Ephesians 3:20 capacity in every area of your life unless you live wholly. Before God can use you to your fullest, He has to work within you completely.

One thing I have learned about leadership is that your capacity to lead is much greater than you can even imagine. You can handle more and do more than you ever comprehended; but unless you are pushed and challenged, you will not realize your capacity.

Just as this is true about leadership, it is true about your whole life. Stop thinking you can only do one thing at a time. Stop settling for less from yourself than you have and you can give. Live up to your capacity!

God has given you the vision and power to live up to your capacity:

- Spiritually: Determine now you are going to take the needed steps to live fit spiritually.
- Physically: Determine now you are going to stop neglecting your physical health and wellness, because God so wills for you to live fit physically.
- Relationally: Determine now you are going to take the needed actions to become healthy relationally, and begin to work diligently to live fit relationally.

- Financially: Determine now to get this part of your life in order and do all you can with all you have to live fit financially.
- Emotionally: Determine now you are going to begin to watch your life gauges more effectively, evaluate yourself more intentionally, and live a grateful life so you can live fit emotionally.

You do have the capacity to monitor and act upon each of these areas of your life simultaneously. With the vision of and by the power of Ephesians 3:20, God can help you live up to your capacity, not just in each of these areas of your life, but wholly.

Take heart my friend. With God on your side, you can do it. Live wholly.

On Your Way to a Healthy You

Living Fit: Make Your Life Count by Pursuing a Healthy You has given you a winning plan that will become an ongoing strategy to true and complete fitness in every area of your life. This strategy is biblical, spiritual, and practical. It is not just a good thing to do, but it is the right thing to do, guaranteeing—as far as it depends on you—you will live a faithful and impactful life.

If you will make this commitment to being fit holistically, it will give you the capacity to become a healthier you. You will not be like an athlete that trains without purpose, but you will be able to declare these words boldly: "So I do not run like the one who runs aimlessly or box like one beating the air" (1 Cor. 9:26). You can hit your stride in this holistic strategy and it will advance your life spiritually, physically, relationally, financially, and emotionally.

I know that I cannot determine how *long* I live, but I can determine *how* I live. Since I want to realize God's vision for my life and expend all I have to seize this vision, I know that the healthier I am in each of these five life areas, the greater my potential to see this vision realized. God has given us the capacity to live out this vision by His power and for His glory.

Speaking of God's power, I believe it is available when you are willing to place your mind, will, emotion, body, and spirit under the Lordship of Jesus Christ and the controlling power of the Holy Spirit daily. Each of us needs to live under His control consistently, regularly, and daily. Approach this strategy as a spiritual calling upon your life. Deal with it spiritually and seriously. Now is the time to get these five areas of your life healthy, both singularly and collectively. When this occurs, the synergy in your life will become a spiritual force like you have not had in a long time, or perhaps you have never had. You will become a healthier you!

> I know that I cannot determine how long I live, but I can determine how I live.

Living Fit is a winning plan. When you are healthy spiritually, physically, relationally, financially, and emotionally, you will be ready to make the biggest impact with your life. You are now on your way to a fit and healthy you.

Your life is a gift from God. You have only one shot with your life. *Make it count!*

Notes

Chapter 2

1. Bruce H. Wilkinson, *The Prayer of Jabez: Breaking Through to the Blessed Life* (Sisters, OR: Multnomah, 2000), 20.

Chapter 7

1. Doyle Rice, "Nearly a Third of World Is Overweight," *USA Today*, June 13, 2017.

Chapter 9

1. *Merriam-Webster*, s.v. "dysfunction," accessed June 2, 2017, https://www.merriam-webster.com/dictionary/dysfunctional.
2. Acts 15.

Chapter 10

1. John 3:16.
2. Hebrews 10:10.
3. Romans 5:8.

Chapter 11

1. W. Oscar Thompson Jr. with Carolyn Thompson, *Concentric Circles of Concern* (Nashville, TN: Broadman Press, 1981), 13.

Chapter 12

1. Thom S. Rainer, *I Am a Church Member* (Nashville, TN: B&H Publishing Group, 2013), 35.

Chapter 13

1. http://www.experian.com/blogs/ask-experian/survey-results-when-divorce-does-damage-to-your-credit/.

2. https://www.bloomberg.com/news/articles/2016-12-15/average-credit-card-debt-16k-total-debt-133k-where-do-you-fit-in.

3. Ibid.

4. Ibid.

5. Ronnie Floyd, interview with Chris Brown, "EP 20: Life and Leadership Today with Guest, Chris Brown," *Life and Leadership Today with Ronnie Floyd,* Podcast audio, July 18, 2017, https://itunes.apple.com/us/podcast/life-and-leadership-today/id1211279930?mt=2.

6. https://www.forbes.com/sites/zackfriedman/2017/02/21/student-loan-debt-statistics-2017/#7c12081a5dab.

7. http://nypost.com/2017/04/16/americans-are-swamped-in-1-trillion-of-credit-card-debt/.

8. http://www.nationaldebtclocks.org/debtclock/unitedstates.

9. https://www.daveramsey.com/askdave/debt/time-to-make-a-life-decision.

10. https://www.daveramsey.com/.

11. Ibid.

12. Ronnie Floyd, interview with Dave Ramsey, *Ronnie Floyd on Life and Leadership Today,* Cross Church, podcast audio, May 16, 2017, http://www.ronniefloyd.com/blog/11706/podcast/ep-11-life-and-leadership-today-with-guest-dave-ramsey/.

13. https://www.daveramsey.com/.

Chapter 14

1. Wallace E. Fisher, *A New Climate for Stewardship* (Nashville, TN: Abingdon, 1976), 28.

Chapter 15

1. 1 Chronicles 29:1-9.

2. Genesis 14:17-20.

3. Matthew 23:23.

4. 2 Corinthians 8.

5. Malachi 3:8–10; Philippians 4:10–20.

6. http://www.boundless.org/faith/2009/the-three-conversions.

Chapter 16

1. *Merriam-Webster*, s.v. "indelible," accessed June 3, 2017, http://www.boundless.org/faith/2009/the-three-conversions.

2. John Maxwell, foreword to book, *The Eternity Portfolio* by Alan Gotthardt (Carol Stream, IL: Tyndale House Publishers, 2003), 13.

Chapter 17

1. Genesis 2:15; Joshua 23:11.

2. Isaiah 62:6.

3. Isaiah 62:7.

4. Hebrews 10:24.

5. Matthew 24:42–44.

6. W. E. Vines, Merrill F. Unger, and William White Jr., *An Expository Dictionary of Biblical Words* (Grand Rapids, MI: Thomas Nelson Publishers, 1984), 206–7.

Chapter 18

1. *Merriam-Webster*, *s.v.* "authentic," accessed June 4, 2017, https://www.merriam-webster.com/dictionary/authentic.

2. James 1:22.

Chapter 20

1. Matthew 7:11f.